OXFORD MEDICAL PUBLICATIONS

HIV and AIDS

PRACTICAL GUIDES FOR GENERAL PRACTICE

HIV and AIDS

MANAGEMENT BY THE PRIMARY CARE TEAM

Practical Guides for General Practice 16

ADRIAN MOSS

General Practitioner, Birmingham and
Adviser to West Midlands Regional Health Authority
HIV Unit

Oxford   New York   Tokyo
OXFORD UNIVERSITY PRESS
1992

Oxford University Press, Walton Street, Oxford OX2 6DP
Oxford New York Toronto
Delhi Bombay Calcutta Madras Karachi
Petaling Jaya Singapore Hong Kong Tokyo
Nairobi Dar es Salaam Cape Town
Melbourne Auckland
and associated companies in
Berlin Ibadan

Oxford is a trade mark of Oxford University Press

Published in the United States
by Oxford University Press, New York

A catalogue record for this book is available from the British Library

Library of Congress Cataloging in Publication Data
Moss, Adrian.
HIV and AIDS: management by the primary care team/Adrian Moss.
(Practical guides for general practice; 16)
(Oxford medical publications)
Includes bibliographical references and index.
1. AIDS (Disease) 2. HIV infections. I. Title. II. Series.
III. Series: Oxford medical publications.
[DNLM: 1. Acquired Immunodeficiency Syndrome—therapy.
2. HIV infections—therapy. 3. Patient Care Team. 4. Primary Health Care.
W1 PR141NK no. 16/WD 308 M913h]
RC607.A26M69 1992   616.97'92—dc20   92-1172
ISBN: 0–19–262216–1 (pbk.)

Typeset by Cotswold Typesetting Limited, Cheltenham
Printed in Great Britain by
Dotesios Ltd, Trowbridge, Wilts.

Preface

There are three important facts that link general practice and HIV disease. Firstly and crucially, HIV infection is preventable. Secondly, HIV causes a chronic disease and those people affected spend the vast majority of their time living in the community. Thirdly, people who have late-stage disease often choose to die in the familiar surroundings of their own home.

For these reasons, HIV-related health care must be provided in the community. Initially, specialized teams provided most of this, but it is increasingly clear that generic services should be the cornerstone of this care. The general practitioner is ideally placed to provide this service because of his or her specialized knowledge and experience of local resources, health promotion, chronic disease, psychological support, and perhaps most importantly, palliative care.

The general practice perspective is essential to the totality of good quality care in HIV disease. This book will give general practitioners the knowledge and confidence to provide that care.

Dr Simon Mansfield
Consultant Physician in Community Liaison, HIV Disease,
Westminster Hospital, London

Acknowledgements

My grateful thanks to Peter Leslie, Tom Matthews, and Mark Cronin of West Midlands Regional Health Authority HIV Unit, for practical support and advice; Dr Ahilya Noone of the CDSC, Colindale, for provision of statistical material; Dr Simon Mansfield, Riverside Health Authority, for encouragement and useful comments; Dr Anthony Pinching of St Mary's Hospital, London, for his sound, sensible, and optimistic views on the subject, which have been an invaluable influence on me over many years; Maria Gomez and Alan Bradley, of World's End Health Centre; Michael Weinstein; and to all my patients, past and present, who have provided unique insight and experience.

Contents

1 Introduction

Background

Experience of AIDS since the disease was first described a decade ago[1,2] appears to have been confined almost entirely to hospital practice. While this has meant that those hospital units with an interest in HIV have developed undoubted skills in diagnosis and management, many GPs feel they lack the knowledge and experience to cope with patients in the community.[3,4]

However most GPs are willing to treat people with HIV infection, and as many as 47 per cent of GPs in some areas have experience of at least one HIV-positive patient.[5] A number of postal surveys between 1988 and 1990, covering several areas of the United Kingdom, demonstrate that, of the 1679 GPs who responded, 34 per cent had patients they knew to be HIV-positive.[3-7]

Furthermore, increasing pressure on hospital services, and the expressed wishes of patients themselves, will increase the trend towards primary care involvement.[8,9]

Few hospital doctors appear to understand either the problems or the opportunities presented in General Practice. Particularly with a new disease such as AIDS, there is a tendency for hospitals to 'hang on' to patients, overlooking the invaluable resources available through the primary care team. This can leave the GP feeling de-skilled and anxious. I believe that as GPs we already have both the willingness, and most of the skills, needed to provide excellent care for those of us in the community affected by HIV.[10]

1

This book aims to outline the basic knowledge required by GPs offering services to people affected by HIV.

Use of language

The use of language is important in an area such as AIDS, as many subjective views are demonstrated by the words we use. In an area where prejudice and misinformation are still common, it is especially important that words are used accurately, with no implication of value judgements.

The term **patient** is used frequently, as most patients seem happy with this term. It is debatable whether someone with HIV who is well should be considered a 'patient', but in the context of dealing with the GP, the term is appropriate.

Person with HIV/AIDS is used in preference to 'victim' or 'sufferer', as many of those affected do not consider themselves to be either victims or sufferers.

People affected by HIV/AIDS is a useful expression, as it includes not only those with the virus, but also their friends, families, and others directly affected.

Gay is used throughout to mean homosexual. 'Homosexual' stresses the sexual aspect too strongly, and is too scientific. The term was first used by nineteenth-century doctors to describe what they believed was an illness. 'Gay', on the other hand, is used by gay people to define themselves, and context always makes the meaning clear. The *Oxford Dictionary* describes the word as 'colloquial': Collins does not, and indeed places 'homosexual' as the first meaning.

The term **drug abuser** has been avoided, as this is a value judgement, and could apply to some GPs with regard to their prescribing!

Case studies

All the people described in this book are real, with only
minor differences of detail which are employed to make a
particular point, or to preserve anonymity. Names have
almost exclusively *not* been changed, as these are **real
people**.

References

1. Du Bois, *et al.* (1981). *Lancet*, **2**, 1339.
2. *Pneumocystis* pneumonia—Los Angeles (1981). *Morbidity and
   Mortality Weekly Reports*, **30**, 250-2.
3. Anderson, P. and Mayon-White (1988). General practitioners and
   management of infection with HIV. *British Medical Journal*, **296**,
   535-7.
4. Sibbald, B. and Freeling, P. (1988). AIDS and the future general
   practitioner. *Journal of the Royal College of General Practitioners*, **38**, 500-2.
5. Roderick, P., Victor, C. R., and Beardrow, R. (1990). Developing
   care in the community: GPs and the HIV epidemic. *AIDS Care*,
   2(2), 127-32.
6. Boyton, R. and Scrambler, G. (1988). Survey of General Practitioners' attitudes to AIDS in the North West Thames and East
   Anglian regions. *British Medical Journal*, **296**, 538-40.
7. Naji, S. A., Russell, I. T., Foy, C. J. W., Gallagher, M., Rhodes, T. J.,
   and Moore, M. P. (1989). HIV infection and Scottish general
   practice: knowledge and attitudes. *Journal of the Royal College
   of General Practitioners*, **39**, 234-8.
8. King, M. (1988). AIDS and the general practitioner: views of
   patients with HIV infection and AIDS. *British Medical Journal*,
   297, 182-4.
9. Mansfield, S. J. and Singh, S. (1989). The general practitioner
   and human immunodeficiency virus infection: an insight into
   patients' attitudes. *Journal of the Royal College of General
   Practitioners*, **39**, 104-5.

10. George, R. and Moss, A. (1991). AIDS–the impact on primary care. In *The medical annual* (ed. J. Fry and T. Bouchier Hayes), pp. 15–21. Clinical Press Ltd, Bristol.

2   What is so special about AIDS?

History and scale of the epidemic

The first report of an acquired immune deficiency syndrome (AIDS) in a British journal was in 1981.[1] In 1983 Barre-Sinoussi and her collegues at the *Institut Pasteur* in Paris discovered the virus associated with AIDS, later named human immunodeficiency virus (HIV). At that time, it appeared that this new disease was affecting certain members of the community specifically, namely haemophiliacs, injecting drug-users, gay men, Haitians, and recipients of blood transfusions. It appeared likely that the infectious agent could be transmitted via blood and blood products and through sexual contact.

The gay community in New York was particularly badly affected, and by 1983, 975 in that city had developed AIDS, 392 of whom had died.[2] About the same time, articles were appearing in Britain about the 'gay plague', and the scene was set for the biggest threat to public health this century.

By the end of 1991, over 1.2 million people world-wide will be living and dying with AIDS, and in Britain 5451 men, women, and children have been diagnosed with the disease, and nearly 17 000 positive HIV antibody tests have

been reported.[3] The number of those known to be infected
has continued to rise dramatically every year, and it is
generally accepted that there are probably four people with
HIV who have not been tested for every one that has. It is
therefore likely that some 85 000 people in this country have
acquired HIV infection. This would give each GP an
average of 3 HIV positive patients.

Preliminary reports from the unlinked anonymous HIV
prevalence monitoring programme in England and Wales[3]
suggest that among male heterosexual attenders at GUM
clinics in London, who were not known to have injected
drugs, prevalence of HIV infection is 1 per cent, and 0.2 per
cent outside London. In Inner London, the prevalence of
HIV infection among pregnant women receiving antenatal
care was 0.19 per cent (1 in 515). As of June 1991, 34 per
cent of people known to have HIV are heterosexual.[4]

The proportion of HIV antibody positive reports in the
sexual intercourse between men and women exposure
category, *which excludes those known to have injected
drugs*, shows a consistent pattern:[3]

Year	1985	1986	1987	1988	1989	1990	1991 (1st qtr)
Proportion	3%	5%	9%	11%	13%	18%	25%

Fear and experience

Why has it taken 10 years for us to accept that this infection
puts *everyone* at risk?

AIDS has brought together all the taboos of modern
society: death, sexuality, drugs, race. To confront AIDS
requires us to confront these taboos, and by and large we
have not been willing to do so.

It is our own fears that cause us constantly to marginalize

those with HIV, by conveniently placing them in 'high-risk groups', rather than considering the *activity* which put them at risk.

This is evident in the presentation of data on those who have acquired HIV. Bisexual men are grouped with gay men, not heterosexuals, and heterosexual contact is divided up according to where the infection was acquired. The result is that the group with the lowest incidence of HIV is exclusively-heterosexual males who have not injected drugs or received blood products, and who have not had sex abroad.

It is frightening for us to accept that we are *all* at risk of HIV, and that it is our *behaviour* that puts us at risk.

However, experience has shown that familiarity with the issues around HIV and AIDS, and particularly direct experience with people with HIV and AIDS, greatly reduces anxiety, and enables effective care to be offered.

The fears surrounding AIDS are understandable, and are common to most of us, as the following situation demonstrates.

In 1984 I was asked to see Clive in hospital. He had no GP, and the ward sister felt I might be able to help. He was thought to have AIDS, and had recently undergone surgery for resection of an area of TB in his bowel. I had never met anyone with AIDS, and was terrified. I had to ring a bell to get into the ward, and eventually found Clive's room. He was sitting up in bed, looking very wasted, with the purple blotches of Kaposi's sarcoma on his face. A nurse was combing his hair, and kissed him as she left. I learnt a great deal from Clive and his nurses—they made a point of touching him, and only wore gloves when taking blood or dealing with body fluids.

My own fears around AIDS diminished with personal experience of the disease. Just as in any other new situation, fear is natural, but diminishes when confronted directly.

What prevents patients with HIV from seeking help from the general practitioner?

- *Perceived lack of confidentiality.* A common fear is that GPs do not respect confidentiality, and that receptionists are less discreet than they should be.[5-7]

- *Unfamiliarity with the practice.* Many people affected by HIV are young, and not used to attending the practice. Some are not registered with a GP at all, and of those who are, about half have not informed the GP of their HIV status.[5,6]

- *Hospitals hang on to patients.* Because this is a new disease, and because many patients are first diagnosed HIV-positive at a GUM clinic, there has been a reluctance for hospitals to encourage patients to use their GPs. Furthermore, many hospital doctors do not understand the function of the GP.

What can we do to remedy this situation?

Some HIV clinics have greatly improved the uptake of GP services by actively encouraging patients to see their GP, or register with one locally.[8] Most keep a list of GPs who are known to be helpful, or who have attended study days on HIV and AIDS. GPs who are keen to help in this area can contact the local clinic health advisers, as well as the FHSA, to inform them of their interest.

It may also be appropriate to inform any local voluntary groups of your willingness to have patients with HIV on your list (see Chapter 18).

Practice leaflets can include information on confidentiality, and may even make a positive statement on policy for dealing with people affected by HIV.

AIDS *is* special—*but not that special!*

References

1. Du Bois *et al.* (1981). *Lancet*, **2**, 1339.
2. Kramer, L. (1990). *Reports from the holocaust*, p. 69. Penguin, London.
3. PHLS AIDS Centre (1991). Unpublished quarterly surveillance tables No. 11.
4. PHLS AIDS Centre (1991). Unpublished press release, June 1991.
5. Mansfield, S. J. and Singh, S. (1989). The general practitioner and human immunodeficiency virus infection: an insight into patients' attitudes. *Journal of the Royal College of General Practitioners*, **39**, 104-5.
6. King, M. B. (1988). AIDS and the general practitioner: views of patients with HIV and AIDS. *British Medical Journal*, **297**, 182-4.
7. King, M. B. (1987). AIDS and the general practitioner: Psycho-social issues. *Health Trends*, **19**, 1-2.
8. Smits, A., Mansfield, S., and Singh, S. (1990). Facilitating care of patients with HIV infection by hospital and primary care teams. *British Medical Journal*, **300**, 241-3.

3 What is so ordinary about AIDS?

Familiar themes

Life-threatening infection associated with sexual activity or the injection of body fluids is not new. We are all familiar with the epidemiology of syphilis and hepatitis B. Treatment for syphilis only became available during this century, and management of hepatitis B is still in its infancy.

As GPs we are also familiar with issues around death and dying, including those where young people are affected. Most of us have experience with other cultures or groups in society, and are used to providing appropriate care.

Confidentiality is second nature to us, and dealing with sensitive issues is a matter of routine.

We are used to co-ordinating a primary care team, so as to provide the most appropriate care for our patients, and we are at least learning about the importance of 'consumer choice', and developing the kind of service people want.

We are used to referring and asking for help when we have problems with a diagnosis or treatment, and we are used to seeing patients with rare diseases, reading them up, and learning from both the patient and the specialist. Indeed in my opinion *we already have the skills required to provide adequate care in the community for those affected by HIV.*[1] We simply have to be prepared to offer these skills to those who need them.

The rest of the primary care team is also well-equipped to meet these needs, as increasing numbers of health care workers are finding.

'Normalization' of HIV and AIDS

In the current climate of fear and prejudice, the importance of confidentiality should never be overlooked; but there is a strong case for working towards the normalization of HIV and AIDS, so that no moral judgements or stigma are applied to those affected. Many individuals with HIV have spoken out about their status, and this has achieved a great deal in raising the awareness of others.

If HIV were seen generally for what it is—a viral infection which can infect anyone, regardless of who they are—the needs of those affected would be better met, and the spread of the epidemic might be limited.

References

1. George, R. and Moss, A. (1991). AIDS—the impact on primary care. In *The medical annual* (ed. J. Fry and T. Bouchier Hayes), pp. 15-21. Clinical Press Ltd, Bristol.

4 Natural history of HIV infection

Human immunodeficiency virus (HIV)

HIV is an RNA virus which possesses an unusual enzyme, *reverse transcriptase*, which allows it to incorporate itself into cellular DNA. The virus has a particular affinity for human T-helper lymphocytes, although it may infect other cells. Having incorporated itself into a host cell, HIV is able to replicate, and may thus eventually severely impair immune function, particularly T-cell-mediated immunity.

Another virus, HIV-2, has now been isolated in a relatively small number of patients. The effects of HIV-2 are similar to those of HIV. In this book, HIV is used to signify the original human immunodeficiency virus, sometimes called HIV-1.

Once HIV has been acquired, it is likely that an individual remains infected, and able to transmit the infection, throughout life, although there are very rare cases of patients who appear to have lost any sign of HIV infection.

The course of HIV infection is extremely variable, and although some may become very ill very quickly, most are well for most of the time. Chronic HIV infection is initially asymptomatic, and in some cases may remain so indefinitely. Indeed, one major study suggests that of those who seroconverted from 1977 to 1980, 19 per cent had not developed signs or symptoms of HIV infection after eight to twelve years.[1]

Classification of HIV infection

No classification is completely adequate, as the course of the diseases related to HIV infection is so variable. There is *not* an inevitable progression from one group to the next.

The American Centers for Disease Control (CDC) have classified HIV infection into four main groups:

Group I: Acute infection

Group II: Asymptomatic infection

Group III: Persistent generalized lymphadenopathy

Group IV: Other diseases, including those infections and tumours which define AIDS, constitutional disease, and other less serious diseases associated with HIV.

Group I–Acute infection

The **seroconversion illness** ranges from a flu-like illness to a meningitis or encephalitis, and may occur up to six weeks after infection; however, it is by no means invariable, and if it does occur it will most often not be recognized as such, either by the patient or the doctor.

Group II–Asymptomatic infection

This group contains patients who show no symptoms or signs of HIV infection. There may or may not be abnormalities in serological tests of immune function.

Group III–Persistent generalized lymphadenopathy (PGL)

Many patients develop **persistent generalized lymphadenopathy (PGL)**, which may be defined as:

enlarged nodes at least 1 cm in diameter in two or more extra-inguinal sites persisting for at least three months, without any current illness or medication known to cause enlarged nodes.

The proportion of patients with PGL who subsequently develop AIDS is 10–30 per cent, but the proportion increases with longer follow-up.[2] However, presence or absence of PGL is not a useful indicator of an individual's likelihood of developing AIDS.

A single very enlarged node should be regarded with suspicion, as lymphoma is relatively common in people with HIV.

Group IV–HIV disease

This group contains a broad spectrum of clinical features related to HIV infection, and may be broadly divided into those which do not define AIDS, and those which do. This is an arbitrary division, which changes from time to time.

HIV disease/AIDS-related complex (ARC)

After some months to some years, an individual may develop clinical symptoms of HIV infection, including constitutional symptoms, such as malaise, fever, anorexia, weight loss; infections, which may be viral (for example shingles), fungal (for example thrush), or bacterial (for example tuberculosis); and oral hairy leukoplakia (see Chapter 7). This group of symptoms and signs is commonly known as 'HIV disease' or 'ARC' (AIDS-related complex).

Patients with this group of conditions are very diverse, and may include some who are very well, for example with minor skin problems, and others who are seriously ill, for example with oral thrush and severe weight loss. However, by definition those who have or who have had an AIDS-defining condition are not included.

The arbitrary nature of any classification of people with HIV is demonstrated by the following example.

Brian came to register with his GP on the advice of the local HIV clinic. He was well, and working at a very busy telephone exchange. His only complaint was of dry, flaky skin on the sides of his nose. The history revealed that an endoscopy some three years previously had shown oesophageal candidiasis, which had responded well to treatment. On examination there was no suggestion of oral thrush.

Since his diagnosis of oesophageal candidiasis, this has been included as an AIDS-defining condition in someone who is HIV-positive. This young man, then, by definition, had AIDS, but was not aware of the fact, simply because of a change in categorization.

In Brian's case, the GP was able to explain the caprices of medical committees and their liking for convenient categories which have more to do with research than individual patients. However, a sensitive explanation was necessary, as another doctor might subsequently have assumed Brian knew he had AIDS.

Acquired immune deficiency syndrome (AIDS)

Certain specified infections and tumours in an individual who is HIV-positive define **AIDS**.

AIDS has been defined as 'a reliably diagnosed disease that is at least moderately indicative of an underlying cellular immune deficiency, in a patient with no known cause of cellular immune deficiency or any other cause of reduced resistance reported to be associated with the disease'.

AIDS-defining infections include *Pneumocystis carinii* pneumonia (the commonest AIDS-defining opportunistic infection in the UK, accounting for about half of all new AIDS diagnoses),[3] cerebral toxoplasmosis, cryptosporidial diarrhoea, and cytomegalovirus infections of the central nervous system, including the eye, the lungs, or the gut. There are many others.

The commonest AIDS-defining tumour is Kaposi's sarcoma, accounting for some 20 per cent of new AIDS diagnoses in the UK.[3]

Prognosis

The number of people with HIV eventually developing AIDS varies from place to place, although the longer the follow-up, the higher the proportion. So far figures vary from 8 per cent in Danish gay men, to 34 per cent among intravenous drug-users in New York.[2] The San Francisco cohort study of gay and bisexual men[1] gives an indication of the probability of developing AIDS:

Years since seroconversion	Percentage developing AIDS
1	0
2	1
3	3
4	8
5	13
6	20
7	28
8	37
9	44
10	51
11	54

Survival with AIDS appears to depend partly upon the presenting disease. About 50 per cent of all AIDS patients survive a little over a year, whereas 50 per cent of white gay males with Kaposi's sarcoma survive just over two years, and about a third of the latter group survive five years and more.[4]

A number of factors have been suggested which affect the prognosis of people with HIV infection. Some of these are discussed in Chapter 9. However it is essential, particularly when counselling patients with HIV, to remember that any figures quoted are statistical, and an individual's progress cannot be predicted accurately.

References

1. Rutherford, G. W., Lifson, A. R., Hessol, N. A., Darrow, W. W., O'Malley, P. M., Buchbinder, S. P., *et al.* (1990). Course of HIV-1 infection in a cohort of homosexual and bisexual men: an 11 year follow up study. *British Medical Journal*, **301**, 1183–8.
2. Adler, M. W. (1987). Care for patients with HIV and AIDS. *British Medical Journal*, **295**, 27–30.
3. Peters, B. S., Beck, E. J., Coleman, D. G., Wadsworth, M. J. H., McGuinness, O., Harris, J. R. W., and Pinching, A. J. (1991). Changing disease patterns in patients with AIDS in a referral centre in the United Kingdom: the changing face of AIDS. *British Medical Journal*, **302**, 203–7.
4. Rothenberg, R., Woelfel, M., Stoneburner, R., Milberg, J., Parker, R., and Truman, B. (1987). Survival with the acquired immune deficiency syndrome. *New England Journal of Medicine*, **317**, 1297–1302.

5   Transmission of HIV

HIV can be detected in most body fluids of an infected individual, but only blood, serum, semen, and vaginal secretions contain the virus in sufficient quantities to transmit infection. It is debatable whether HIV can be transmitted through breast milk; but vertical transmission *in utero* and possibly during birth occurs in about 13 per cent of cases.[1] Donated semen and organs can also transmit the virus.

Factors affecting the transmission of HIV include the infectivity of the individual (infectivity is probably highest in the weeks following infection, when there is no detectable HIV AB, and in those with AIDS); the degree of exposure; presence of trauma or secondary infection; and the presence of epithelial receptors for HIV.[2]

It follows that behaviour allowing transmission of HIV includes:

- **sexual intercourse (active or passive, heterosexual or gay)**
- **parenteral injection**
- **receipt of donated organs or semen**
- **possibly breast-feeding**

To this list should be added any sexual or other activity where there is a chance of infected blood, serum, semen, or vaginal fluid entering the body.

In practice, by far the commonest routes of transmission are unprotected sexual intercourse and parenteral injection of infected blood or serum.

At the beginning of the epidemic, it appeared that certain **groups** were at particular risk of HIV infection, namely haemophiliacs, recipients of blood transfusions, Haitians, gay men, and injecting drug-users. To this list were later added prostitutes, central Africans, and those who had had sex with any of the above. However it is now clear that it is not membership of a group that increases risk, but **behaviour**.

The notion of **risk groups** is fatally flawed. It allows those who do not belong to any of these groups to feel falsely secure, and it encourages severe discrimination against those who do belong to these groups. The truth is that we are all at risk of HIV infection—it is our **behaviour** that puts us at risk. The other fallacy is that society is made up of distinct groups. This is clearly a false notion—some haemophiliacs are injecting drug-users: some injecting drug-users are gay.

Assessment of risk

In practice, how can you assess an individual's risk of having HIV infection?

The truth is that it is impossible. There are some who have acquired HIV infection through unprotected intercourse once or twice with an infected partner. Others have had multiple partners over many years, many of whom are HIV-positive, without becoming infected. A clear history of repeated high-risk activity is certainly an indication that the individual may have acquired HIV, and absence of any high-risk behaviour should indicate no risk of having the virus. But between these two extremes it is impossible to assess risk.

What about the sexual partners of those at particular risk? It must be assumed that they too may have acquired HIV infection—indeed, as time goes by, there may be very few people who have *never* been at risk of HIV infection.

This is a sobering thought, and should leave us all feeling a little uncomfortable. The recent results from random anonymous screening have shown that the overall prevalence of HIV infection among women attending antenatal clinics in inner London is one in five hundred, with one in two hundred in some clinics.[3] In two London GUM clinics, one in ninety-one heterosexual men were HIV+. In New York, AIDS has for some years been the commonest cause of death among young men, and is now the commonest cause of death among young women.

Unless we all understand and practice safe behaviour, the current epidemic will not stop, and we shall be facing the biggest threat to public health we have ever experienced.

However, increasing numbers of patients clearly *do* understand the threat of HIV and AIDS, and GPs are increasingly being asked for advice in this area.

Jill has come to see you very distressed. She has been going out with John for three years, and they are seriously considering getting married.

You see from her records that she has been on the pill for about three years, and she's had two normal cervical smears. John has never made any secret about his previous girlfriends, but he has now told Jill that before he met her he had sex with a number of women over a period of some years, so he has decided to have an HIV antibody test. Jill is now terrified in case she has AIDS.

This situation is likely to occur with increasing frequency, and can be difficult to handle. There is no doubt that by having unprotected sexual intercourse, Jill has been at risk of acquiring HIV. She may want to wait until John has his test result, and she may decide that she wants an HIV antibody test herself. If so, all the implications of this should be fully disucussed (see Chapter 6). Some GPs may prefer to refer Jill to the local GUM clinic, where appropriate counselling will be available. On the other hand, some GPs may feel that in reality the risk that Jill is HIV-positive is so small that basic reassurance is all that is required. In any case, it should be possible, with a careful history and examination, to reassure Jill that she does not have AIDS.

Social contact

There is absolutely no evidence that HIV can be trans-mitted through day-to-day social contact, either person-to-person or through objects such as cutlery, cups, and plates. In theory the virus could be transmitted through shared use of razors or toothbrushes, particularly if there is fresh blood on these objects; but in practice this has never been demonstrated, and in any case, normal hygiene would inhibit most people from sharing these.

Intimate bodily contact where there is no exchange of potentially infected body fluids cannot transmit HIV. So we should all be reassured that hugging, kissing, cuddling, and touching others present no risk whatsoever.

Clinical contact

In the UK there has been one reported case of a health worker possibly acquiring HIV infection through a needle-stick injury while resheathing a needle; but follow-up of 125 infected blood inoculation injuries in this country revealed not one single seroconversion.

It is sensible to cover all cuts with elastoplast, and to wear latex gloves whenever there is risk of contact with blood, or body fluids that are visibly contaminated with blood.

In the clinical setting, there is no substitute for the use of sensible practices for the prevention of cross-infection. It is false to assume that by using extra precautions with individuals who are HIV-positive, or with those deemed to have been at particular risk, the risk of transmission can be minimized.

Safe behaviour

Safe behaviour may be defined as the avoidance by an individual of any activity which puts him or her at risk of acquiring or transmitting HIV infection.

Following this definition, safe behaviour applies as much to the health care worker as to the patient. Good clinical practice is as important in the prevention of HIV infection as safe sex.

As everyone is at risk of HIV infection, it is appropriate for the GP and the practice nurse to use every opportunity to educate the public about safe behaviour. Any family planning advice should include information about this (many patients think that the 'protection' provided by the pill provides protection against sexually transmitted diseases); and there are many other scenarios where it is appropriate to discuss safe behaviour.

In my practice we marked the patient summary card every time safe behaviour was discussed, as this avoids unnecessary repetition.

Health promotion clinics can be used to promote safe behaviour. While many patients would be embarrassed to attend an identified safe behaviour clinic, information can be included in many other clinics, such as travel clinics and well person clinics.

Safe behaviour advice should include information on:

- safe sex (correct use of condoms/spermicides) for the sexually active
- use of clean needles and syringes for injecting drug-users
- correct clinical practice for those in contact with body fluids.

Condoms

A number of studies have shown the effectiveness of condoms in reducing the rate of transmission of HIV; however, there is a failure rate in preventing pregnancy, through misuse or rupture, of 0.6–14.7 per 100 woman years.[4] It is therefore essential that correct use of condoms is explained to patients by the GP, the practice nurse, or the family planning worker.

If a lubricant is used with a condom it should be water-based, to prevent damage to the latex. Lubricants containing a spermicide, for example nonoxynol-9, may offer added protection against the transmission of HIV, as spermicides can inactivate HIV *in vitro.*

The patient should understand that the condom must be worn whenever there is contact with the other person, as prostatic fluid may contain HIV: and the condom should be held carefully on the penis during withdrawal.

Oral sex

Repeated receptive oral sex has been associated with seroconversion in women in one study,[5] although others dispute this. For those who enjoy oral sex, it is best to explain that there is evidence of possible transmission of HIV, and that ideally a condom should be worn. In any case, it is best to stop short of ejaculation.

References

1. European collaborative study (1991). Children born to women with HIV infection: natural history and risk of transmission. *Lancet,* **337**, 253–60.
2. Adler, M. W. (1987). Care for patients with HIV infection and AIDS. *British Medical Journal,* **295**, 27–30.
3. Communicable disease report (1991). PHLS. Vol. 1, review no. 7.
4. Vessey *et al.* (1988). Factors influencing use-effectiveness of the condom. *British Journal of Family Planning,* **14**, 40–3.
5. Fischl, M. and Dickinson, G. (1987). Women with AIDS in Miami. Abstract WP91. Third international conference on AIDS, Washington DC.

6 HIV antibody testing

Introduction

There is a vital need to recognize that the counsellor in HIV must remain a person offering a trusting, implicitly and explicitly supportive, ongoing and confidential relationship that rises above the rhetoric, the hype, the unrealistic expectations and the hidden agendas embraced by the public discussions to which they, and their patients, are perpetually exposed, whatever their profession.[1]

What the test is

A positive HIV antibody test indicates that an individual has been infected with HIV. Seroconversion usually occurs some six weeks to three months following exposure, although very rarely it can take much longer.

The standard test for HIV antibody in Britain is an ELISA enzyme-linked assay, and if this is positive, the laboratory will arrange a further assay, usually the Western blot, using the same serum sample. The false positive rate following these two tests is negligible.

Results are returned after about two weeks, but in practice a negative result is likely to arrive earlier than a positive result, which is normally re-tested.

What HIV antibody positive means

A positive HIV antibody result gives no indication when the individual was exposed to the virus, and gives no information about infectivity or prognosis, nor does it give any indication at all about the degree of immune deficiency, if any.

It is prudent to assume that anyone with a positive HIV antibody result is potentially infectious for the rest of their lives.

Many patients think the antibody test is 'a test for AIDS'. Indeed the media still persist in using the term 'AIDS test', but it is important to make it clear that a positive HIV antibody test merely indicates that the individual has been exposed to HIV and is infected.

There is one exception. A neonate may acquire HIV antibody from the mother. This may persist for up to two years, and does not necessarily indicate that the child is infected with HIV. Clinical factors and other tests are required to determine whether the child is actually infected (see Chapter 13).

What HIV antibody negative means

A negative HIV antibody result indicates only that the individual has no detectable antibody to HIV. It normally takes up to three months to develop antibody following infection with the virus, so a negative antibody result is not proof of freedom from infection. Rarely, antibody may take much longer to develop, and may indeed never be detectable—and in a few individuals with HIV, the antibody may disappear.

If an individual is considered to have been at risk of infection with HIV, most authorities would recommend two HIV antibody tests three months apart; if these are both negative, it is extremely unlikely that there is HIV infection. However, if there has been additional risk of exposure between the two tests, it would be advisable to arrange another test after a further three months.

Some patients request a certificate of freedom from HIV infection, either for their own personal use, or for a third party such as a foreign consulate in order to obtain a visa. In this case it is essential to make clear on your report that the individual has had an HIV antibody test on that date, which was negative. It is not accurate to state that he or she is not infected with HIV.

Pre-test counselling

It is essential that anyone undergoing an HIV antibody test for any reason should understand what the test is for, and what it means and does not mean. They should also understand the implications of actually having the test, and it should be made clear what will happen to the result.

Many clinics now ask the patient to sign a statement confirming that the meaning of the test has been explained, and that they understand what it means. This may not be appropriate in general practice; but in some cases it should be considered. Because of the serious implications of merely having an HIV antibody test, whatever the result, it is essential that the patient should be fully informed.

There are still unfortunate cases where patients have been tested for HIV antibody without properly understanding what the test means, and even without their knowledge. This can cause untold stress, and can destroy a patient's trust in the medical profession. There have been many arguments about situations in which a patient may be HIV tested without consent—for example if urgent surgery is needed and the patient is unconscious. Universal precautions would obviate the need for this.

There is something of a trend towards more directive counselling than in the past, in view of the improvements in management of patients with HIV. Many experts argue that intervention can be offered earlier, and diagnoses made earlier if patients know they are HIV-positive—and that the stress in finding out they are positive is better handled when well than when seriously ill. It does appear that those presenting late, and untested, do worse than others. There is also the argument that safe behaviour is more likely to be practised if patients know they are HIV-positive.

Anyone offering pre-test counselling should ask the following questions:

- Why are the patients considering a test?
- What risks do they feel they have been at?
- Do they understand the meaning of the test?
- How will they react if it's positive?
- How will they react if it's negative?
- Whom will they tell about the result?
- What do they want to do with the result?
- What support do they have?
- Have they considered the implications for insurance companies, employers, etc.?

In vew of the time needed to go through all these points, and the many implications, many GPs feel happier referring the patient to the GUM clinic. This also avoids the problem with insurance companies. However, if a patient has felt confident enough to come to you to discuss having a test, it is appropriate that you should be informed, and involved in any follow-up.

The serious question of confidentiality should be examined carefully, and is dealt with in Chapter 10. However, it is at this stage that the matter of what you do with the result is likely to be raised, and it is important to have a clear policy.

My view is that our first job is to provide care for our patients, and any other considerations are secondary. Some patients want to have an 'off the record' discussion about HIV, and if they want no record of this to appear in their notes, they have every right to demand this.

Completing the request form

Most GPs have direct access to a laboratory which will perform HIV antibody testing, and many laboratories have a specific request form. In some areas testing is only done at the local GUM clinic, in which case a brief letter of introduction is useful for the clinic and the patient, and should ensure that the GP gets the result.

The HIV antibody request form, apart from the usual patient details, will often ask for specific risk activity. This has been considered useful as it provides epidemiological data, although it is debatable how useful the concept of 'risk group' is, as society is so diverse.

Some patients are quite happy to have their name printed on the form; others prefer anonymity, and in this case it is best to use a pseudonym (I normally ask the patient to suggest one) or a code. The important thing is to keep a record of the name or code used, so that the patient can be informed of the result.

If you are not used to requesting this test, it is helpful to speak to the laboratory, who will clarify any problems.

When the blood is taken at the surgery, it is prudent to ensure that any details on the form are not visible, in order to maintain confidentiality.

Post-test counselling

Every patient should be given a follow-up appointment at which the result of the test can be discussed. This is essential, as there are specific considerations, whatever the result.

● *Negative result*

It should be reiterated that this means that there is no evidence of HIV infection, but that if there has been exposure to risk in the last three months another test is advisable. It should also be made clear that future risk activity still places the individual at risk of infection.

Patients who, in spite of a negative result, keep requesting further tests, have been classed as the 'worried well', and they present particular problems. The worried well are discussed in Chapter 11.

● *Positive result*

At this point it is useful to take a full medical history, and examine the patient, if this has not already been done, as, in the absence of any symptoms or signs of HIV infection, it is possible to reassure patients that, even though they have HIV infection, there is no sign whatsoever that any damage has been done to the immune system (see Chapter 7).

Some patients may appear totally unsurprised at the result, and this may indeed be evidence that they did seriously consider they had HIV infection. None the less, it is still important to explore any anxieties they have, and provide strong reassurance where possible.

The matter of support should be discussed fully, as the initial shock can cause significant distress. It is a good idea to make clear to patients that they can call you for advice at any time, and to provide a list of contact numbers where help will be available. Health advisers at GUM clinics are generally very helpful, and there are a number of local and national voluntary agencies that provide telephone and face-to-face counselling and other support.

The question of 'whom to tell' should be raised directly. Some patients immediately tell a number of friends and relatives, only to find that those they have confided in need support, or that there is an unfavourable reaction. It is helpful to have one or two friends who can be told, if it is felt their reaction will be favourable; but it is wise to keep the information relatively private until the issues have been examined carefully.

Should you now refer the patient to hospital? The matter of referring a sick patient is discussed in Chapter 7. For those with no symptoms or signs of immune deficiency, a decision can be taken by the patient and yourself.

There is still much controversy about the wisdom of intervention with drugs in someone with HIV who is well. However, intervention is not purely a matter of drugs, and clinics with experience of patients with HIV can provide a great deal of support with counselling and dietary and lifestyle advice, as well as monitoring clinical and laboratory measures of immune function.

None the less, some patients prefer not to be seen at the hospital, and are more comfortable attending the practice, and if the GP is happy to provide a service this is perfectly acceptable. In most cases there can be a happy compromise, where there is 'shared care', with the patient attending a clinic occasionally, and the GP at other times. As in any situation, this only works effectively if there is communication between hospital and GP. Communication is discussed in Chapter 10.

Conclusions

- HIV antibody testing should only be offered by a GP who fully understands the meaning of the test and its implications for the patient.
- Testing should only be with the informed consent of the patient.
- The patient must know what will happen to the result.

- Every patient should be given the result personally at a follow-up appointment, whatever the result.
- If the test is positive, arrangements for support must be made immediately.

References

1. Miller, D. and Pinching, A. (1989). HIV tests and counselling: current issues. *AIDS*, **3** (suppl. 1), S187–S193.

7   Clinical aspects

History-taking

As in any consultation in General Practice, it is important to obtain an accurate picture of the events that have led the patient to consult you, and to clarify by direct questioning any symptoms that will help in formulating a diagnosis.

A great advantage in General Practice is that the patient is probably known to you or the team already, so that rapport may be quickly established and history-taking is considerably shortened. Furthermore, you should be able to formulate a 'whole view' of the patient in a way that is rarely possible in hospital practice, as you already know the patient; you have experience of General Practice; and the patient is likely to be more relaxed in the familiar surroundings of the practice.

There are three groups of patients who may consult you about HIV-related problems—those who know they are HIV-positive, those who have not been tested and who have no signs of HIV disease, and those who are untested but who do have signs of HIV disease.

Known HIV-positive

This is the most straightforward group, as you can address directly the question of whether the presenting problem is HIV-related or not. It is helpful to ask patients whether they feel their symptoms are related to HIV, as you will probably be voicing their fears directly, and these can then be tackled effectively. Your history-taking should include important symptoms of HIV disease, which will give you an impression of the degree, if any, of immune deficiency, and alert you to the likelihood of a serious opportunistic infection which needs urgent intervention.

Unknown status, asymptomatic

This group will contain the 'worried well', who are not HIV-positive but fear they may be, and those who are HIV-positive but have not been tested, including some who consider they may be HIV-positive, and others who consider this unlikely or unthinkable.

The 'worried well' are discussed in Chapter 11, as they present a particular problem for the GP.

Those who consider they may be HIV-positive can be approached in a positive way, similarly to those who know they are HIV-positive. The presenting problems can be dealt with frankly, and the patient's fears about HIV can be discussed openly. It is again a matter of eliciting symptoms that may be attributable to HIV, and following these up appropriately.

Unknown status, symptomatic

The most difficult group is those who show symptoms or signs suggestive of HIV disease, but who have either not considered or rejected the idea that they may have HIV. The GP is here once again in the favourable position of knowing the patients and their circumstances. The approach here depends entirely on the situation, but if there appear to be symptoms and signs of a serious opportunistic infection, it is usually appropriate to raise the question of HIV, while explaining that many infections are readily treated.

In the real world, the GP has to cope with situations that are not simple and clear-cut, and which rarely appear in textbooks. Patients too, thank goodness, rarely fit into neat social and diagnostic groups. This is the challenge of general practice.

When considering the possibility of HIV infection, the first thing is to think of it. The so-called 'risk groups' are increasingly irrelevant to the assessment of an individual's likelihood of being HIV-positive. A better approach may be to ask directly whether the patient has personal experience of anyone with HIV; but if it is appropriate to find out about specific risk behaviour, ask directly: I have never had an angry response from a non-judgemental request for information. For example, 'Have you ever injected drugs?' or 'Have you ever had sex with another man?' These questions need be no more threatening than 'Have you ever had a blood transfusion?' This information may be important, but will rarely be offered unless the questions are asked. Reassurance about confidentiality is essential here, and this is discussed in Chapter 10.

It is important to stress that no amount of conjecture can tell you whether a patient is HIV-positive or not. One gay man with vast and recent unprotected sexual experience with men all over the USA and Europe was repeatedly

HIV-negative: a woman who had had unprotected sex with her one boyfriend was HIV-positive.

Having decided that you are or may be dealing with someone who has HIV, what should you be particularly alert for in the history?

Symptoms to ask about

- **Constitutional symptoms**, particularly over a period exceeding a few days, may be due to HIV disease. These include unaccustomed fatigue or tiredness, malaise, anorexia, weight loss, and fever and sweats (particularly if severe enough to require changing pillows or sheets).

- **Skin complaints** are common, including seborrhoeic dermatitis, eczema, folliculitis, *Herpes simplex*, and fungal infections, including those affecting the nails. However these are common among those without HIV infection. On the other hand, *Herpes zoster* and oral thrush in an individual not otherwise predisposed (as are for example the elderly, those with diabetes, and those undergoing immunosuppressive therapy) are suggestive of HIV infection.

- A patient may present with the purple lesions of **Kaposi's sarcoma** (see below).

- **Gastrointestinal symptoms** are common in HIV disease, but are often rather non-specific, with occasional mild diarrhoea, often over a period of several months.

- **Respiratory symptoms** must always be asked about, as *Pneumocystis carinii* pneumonia (PCP) is a common and treatable opportunistic infection (OI) (see below).

- **Central nervous system symptoms** include headache, visual disturbance (scotoma, blurred vision), paraesthesiae, vomiting, and fits.

● **Previous history.** Ask about oral thrush and shingles.

Examination

Does the patient look unwell? This may sound fatuous, but experience shows that virtually no-one with serious HIV-disease feels well and looks well.

There are three important signs which are virtually pathognomonic of HIV disease:

1. *Oral hairy leukoplakia.* This is a white, adherent plaque, with a furry, or 'hairy' appearance, on the sides of the tongue or underneath it, or on the buccal mucosa. It is readily distinguished from plaques of thrush, as it does not scrape off with a spatula. Usually there are no symptoms, although occasionally the patient may complain of pain or soreness in the area.

The lesion is probably of no prognostic significance, but indicates HIV infection with a very high degree of probability.

2. *Oral thrush.* Excluding patients with precipitating factors—for example the elderly, diabetics, and those on immunosuppressive therapy or antibiotics—this is a good indicator that the patient has HIV infection, and indeed that there is at the time of examination sufficient immuno-deficiency to allow overgrowth of *Candida*. The plaques may be single, multiple, or confluent, usually on the hard or soft palate and on the buccal mucosa, and may be readily scraped off with a spatula. The patient may or may not complain of soreness or a feeling of furriness in the mouth or throat.

A white or discoloured coating on the tongue is not a useful sign, as it is so common, and a mouth or throat swab which shows *Candida albicans* is often of no significance, as this organism is a common commensal.

The importance of oral thrush is that it gives a clue to possible HIV infection, it shows that there is a degree of immune deficiency, and it is readily treated. If a patient presents with oral thrush and has not recently been seen at the clinic, it is better to arrange this than simply to treat the thrush, as it is such a useful marker of immune function.

3. **_Kaposi's sarcoma (KS)._** This is described below. It does occur in certain populations unassociated with HIV infection; but in a patient who is HIV-positive it is an AIDS-defining condition.

It is important to stress that KS is often found in an individual with HIV who is otherwise perfectly well; that on its own it has the best prognosis among AIDS-defining conditions; and that it is eminently responsive to a number of treatments. However, the lesions are usually not painful, and the main reason for intervention would be cosmetic.

Other skin problems have been listed above, but are very common in the population as a whole, so that it is difficult to draw conclusions from them about an individual's immune function.

Treatment for skin conditions is routine, but may need to be persistent. The main proviso would be to avoid strong topical steroids for any length of time, owing to the risk of systemic absorption.

David is 59 and has only attended surgery previously for attention to his ear wax. He looks and feels exceedingly well, but is a little concerned about some 'pimples' on his skin. He is gay, having lived with his lover for over thirty years.

Examination reveals a dozen or so typical umbilicated lesions of _Molluscum contagiosum_ on his face and trunk, but on one shoulder and on his hard palate are two purple lesions of about 3 mm, which do not blanch, and appear typical of Kaposi's sarcoma.

Fundi should be examined frequently, particularly if there is clinical immune deficiency, as cytomegalovirus (CMV) retinitis is not uncommon in people with AIDS, and can be treated. Examination reveals vascular narrowing, irregularity, and occlusion, then perivascular exudates and haemorrhage. Anyone with retinal change should be referred immediately.

Presentations of AIDS

We shall now consider three common presentations of AIDS, which are significant because of their frequency and amenability to treatment.

Kaposi's sarcoma

This is an endothelial tumour which may present in an HIV-positive patient who is otherwise well, or may be found incidentally in others with AIDS. In the HIV-positive patient it is an AIDS-defining condition.

The lesion or lesions are typically pink to purple in colour and from less than a millimetre to several centimetres across, and may develop on any part of the skin or mucous membranes, as well as in other organs. The lesions are usually flat, or may be raised slightly, and are not painful initially. They do not blanch on pressure, and this is a very useful sign, as any coloured lesion that *does* blanch is *not* Kaposi's sarcoma. Diagnosis can only be made by biopsy, but this should only be offered if the result will affect management.

The lesions do not metastasize, although multiple primaries may develop.

Treatment is frequently not necessary, but may be offered for cosmetic reasons, and is highly effective. Low-dose chemotherapy or radiotherapy are particularly effective, with minimal, if any, side-effects.

Pneumocystis carinii pneumonia

This is the commonest presentation of AIDS in the UK, and is due to the protozoon *Pneumocystis carinii*, which is ubiquitous in the environment and in the lungs. Severe immune deficiency or malnutrition allow the organism to multiply in the lungs, gradually filling them with pneumocysts, but with little inflammatory response, so that fever may be absent.

The patient is unwell, and on careful questioning, will describe several weeks' increasing shortness of breath on exertion, with a dry or barely productive cough. Some patients describe a feeling of being unable to get enough breath into the lungs. Shortness of breath can be rather subjective, but is significant if noticed when walking, particularly uphill, with a fit companion who does not become short of breath.

These symptoms must be carefully elicited, as they can be of very insidious onset, and those with (and those who are afraid they may have) HIV may be too frightened of PCP to admit to them readily.

Examination may reveal weight loss or other signs of HIV disease (oral hairy leukoplakia, oral thrush, Kaposi's sarcoma); fever may or may not be present; and chest signs are frequently normal. However, tachypnoea is usual.

Chest X-ray may show a perihilar haze, which progresses to diffuse symmetrical shadowing of the mid- and lower zones with peripheral sparing. However, very often the appearances are normal. Normal sputum culture does not assist diagnosis. However, blood gases show hypoxia, and this is the most useful test for making a diagnosis.

The GP should refer immediately any HIV-positive patient with malaise, cough, and dyspnoea, even in the absence of clinical signs and with a normal chest radiograph. In the less unwell patient, with minimal symptoms, early review may be appropriate, possibly with an anti-biotic—but *not* co-trimoxazole, as this is useful in the treatment of PCP, and may delay diagnosis. Some patients with PCP look deceptively well, tanned if they have recently been abroad or under the sun lamp, and not obviously short of breath if they have been sitting for a while before you see them. James is a good example of this.

James had never been tested for HIV antibody, although he considered he had been at some risk in the past. His GP knew he was gay, but when James presented with a dry cough and a little dyspnoea he looked so well it seemed appropriate to prescribe a course of erythromycin. Three weeks later, it was evident that he had lost weight, and the cough and dyspnoea were worse. A deputizing doctor was called in over the weekend, and, presumably taken in by the tanned, panting patient, who was eager to minimize his symptoms, diagnosed anxiety, and prescribed diazepam.

The next day, James's lover was worried enough to call in a GP with experience of HIV disease, who was immediately struck by the dyspnoea and tachypnoea, evident on walking a few yards on level ground. On examination, there were a few flecks of *Candida* in his mouth, and a small patch of oral hairy leukoplakia. Chest sounds were normal. Immediate admission was arranged.

Diagnosis of PCP is made by demonstration of *P. carinii* on bronchoscopy or induced sputum; but treatment is often started before final diagnosis.

Treatment is with oral or intravenous co-trimoxazole, pentamidine, or a number of other antibiotics, and is highly effective, particularly if an early diagnosis is made. At one centre, PCP accounted for 46 per cent of known causes of death in 1986, but only 3 per cent in 1989.[1]

If the patient is evidently dyspnoeic, most authorities would recommend immediate treatment with intravenous co-trimoxazole or pentamidine. If blood gases reveal a PO_2 below 8, corticosteroids should be considered, as the prognosis is more likely to be unfavourable.

There is increasing evidence that prophylaxis against PCP is effective—most patients who have recovered from the first episode are now offered fortnightly nebulized pentamidine, daily or less frequent co-trimoxazole, or weekly dapsone and pyrimethamine; and some centres advise primary prophylaxis to those with significant loss of immune function. Prophylaxis against PCP is discussed more fully in Chapter 8.

Even a GP experienced in HIV disease may be fooled into missing a diagnosis of PCP. The following describes one such incident.

Chris had attended his GP from time to time with minor skin problems, and had discussed the possibility of HIV infection. However, he felt he would not cope well if he knew he had the virus, though he assumed that he might have it.

He came to surgery with a persistent cough following a minor upper respiratory tract infection, but denied any dyspnoea or malaise. He had scattered rhonchi in his chest, and was keen to try a salbutamol inhaler—and indeed this eased his symptoms. Two weeks later he returned with a worsening cough, but refused to consider any investigation for PCP, and was given an antibiotic.

After a few days the GP was called in to see him at home. He was severely distressed and had lost weight, and his cough was worse. He was weak, and very short of breath on the least exertion. The GP eventually persuaded him to be seen at the local HIV clinic, where blood gases showed severe hypoxia, and he was admitted for treatment of PCP. Despite aggressive therapy with co-trimoxazole and then pentamidine his hypoxia increased, and he became very confused. Eventually he was started on clindamycin, and after three weeks was fit enough to be discharged. Two months later he was able to return to full-time work.

Pyrexia of unknown origin

There are a number of opportunistic infections that may present as pyrexia of unknown origin in a patient with immune deficiency. Many of these are treatable, so while it is often difficult for the GP to make a precise diagnosis, it is important to make an urgent referral.

The patient with known HIV infection and consequent immune deficiency will often show features of significant immune deficiency, such as malaise, weight loss, and oral thrush. There may already be a formal AIDS diagnosis. It is unusual for serious opportunistic infection to present in the absence of these features.

Symptoms may point to the system affected, for example diarrhoea, cough, headache, or confusion. Any features of neurological disease would favour immediate referral, as would any infection in a seriously debilitated or rapidly deteriorating patient. The only exception would be the patient who wants to remain at home, and is happy to forgo the potential benefits of a firm diagnosis.

The situation with a patient not known to have HIV infection is more difficult; however, a careful history may give some clues. There are usually signs of HIV disease, which greatly help in making a diagnosis: oral hairy leukoplakia, oral thrush, and possibly Kaposi's sarcoma. In any case, the patient is usually ill enough for most GPs to consider referral regardless of diagnosis.

Dennis had been treated for pulmonary tuberculosis three years earlier, and at that time was found to have HIV infection. He had remained well until a few weeks ago, when oral thrush became troublesome; but this responded well to oral ketoconazole. The GP was called in because Dennis appeared to have 'flu and was confined to his bed.

He was lying in a darkened bedroom, rather drowsy and a little confused. He had lost weight, and examination revealed a few plaques of thrush in his mouth, and two lesions on the palate suggestive of Kaposi's sarcoma. His temperature was 38.5°C. There were no chest signs, and there was no neck stiffness, but there was right-sided weakness, with an upgoing plantar reflex on the right.

Immediate admission was arranged. A CT scan suggested cerebral toxoplasmosis, and he was treated urgently with Fansidar®, responding so well that he was discharged ten days later.

Referral

The arrangements for the hospital care of patients with HIV vary from place to place, normally involving the genito-urinary medicine or haemophilia clinic and a number of consultants. However, the systems affected by HIV are so numerous that there is often a case to be made for referring to the specialist in the appropriate field, as for example in the case of a diabetic patient with visual problems, whom the GP may choose to refer to an ophthalmologist rather than to the diabetic physician. Lisa's case is an example.

Lisa had remained well with HIV, although she was troubled by severe genital herpes. She was on zidovudine, and was very active. Her mother called the GP in as she had become very weak over the last few days, and was now unable to get up from the toilet without assistance.

Arriving at the house, the GP found Lisa lying in bed looking unwell. She had some proximal muscle wasting and tenderness, but no other significant clinical signs. He felt she had some strange viral illness; but, as the problems were apparently neurological, referred her to the consultant neurologist, who admitted her the same day.

The neurologist diagnosed a toxic reaction to zidovudine, and on cessation of the drug she made a full recovery.

It is possible that the genito-urinary physicians who normally treated Lisa would have considered zidovudine toxicity; but her prompt management by the neurologist could not have been better, and the neurology team gained useful experience.

Conclusions

History and examination can often quickly determine that patients have HIV disease, even if their HIV antibody statuses are unknown. This is not complicated or difficult, and the alert GP, even without any experience of HIV disease, is unlikely to miss the following significant features.

Previous history: risky behaviour, shingles.

Current symptoms: malaise, sweats, cough, dyspnoea, visual disturbance.

Examination: oral thrush, oral hairy leukoplakia, Kaposi's sarcoma, fundal changes.

References

1. Peters, B. S., Beck, E. J., Coleman, D. G., Wadsworth, M. J. H., McGuinness, O., Harris, J. R. W., and Pinching, A. J. (1991). Changing disease patterns in patients with AIDS in a referral centre in the United Kingdom: the changing face of AIDS. *British Medical Journal*, **302**, 203-7.

8 Laboratory investigations

Introduction

Routine laboratory investigations should be performed on the HIV positive patient in just the same way as for any other, according to the specific indications. Forms and bottles should have a biohazard warning sticker, and this may have to be explained to the patient. Some laboratories are reluctant to perform certain tests on high-risk samples, so for less common tests it may be helpful to speak to the laboratory.

There are now some tests for immune function which are available to GPs in a few areas, although they are used mostly by hospitals. However patients often ask about the meaning of any results they have been given—indeed some attach great importance to them—so it is useful to know something about them.

T-helper/CD4+ cell count

T-helper or CD4+ count is a quantitative measure of the lymphocytes to which HIV binds specifically, and which may become depleted as a result of HIV infection. T-helper count varies enormously among individuals, and in an individual from day to day and from hour to hour. However, most authorities agree that a count *repeatedly* under 400 in an HIV-positive patient is an indication of immune deficiency, even in the absence of clinical signs. A result under 200 is generally taken as an indication of marked immune deficiency, with an increased risk of development of AIDS.

43

With a count persistently below 200 most specialists would recommend an anti-retroviral drug and PCP prophylaxis.

HIV antigen/p24 antigen

HIV antigen or p24 antigen measures the amount of circulating viral protein. This is normally negative for most of the course of HIV infection, but some individuals may have detectable viral antigen at various times, and this is of doubtful significance. However a persistently raised HIV antigen, particularly if the titre is rising, may indicate deteriorating immune function, and carries an increased risk of developing AIDS. Some would recommend that in this situation anti-retroviral and PCP-prophylactic treatment should be considered.

Interpretation of results

With both these laboratory tests, it is important to remember that they are only of statistical importance—there are patients with T-helper counts of below 200 who are well, with no signs of immune deficiency, and some who develop AIDS with a count of over 400. Equally, some with repeatedly positive HIV Ag appear to remain well, while a review of patients admitted to the Westminster hospital with AIDS showed that one-third were HIV Ag negative (personal communication).

On the other hand, for those with a T-helper count below 200, there is a 30 per cent risk of developing PCP within one year.[1]

Any interpretation of these test results should be made in the context of the patient. Someone who has no symptoms, and no signs of HIV disease, but a low T-helper count and raised HIV Ag, may not require any intervention; whereas someone with the same results, but with constitutional illness, oral thrush, and other signs of immune deficiency clearly has immunological damage, and would probably benefit from anti-retroviral therapy and PCP prophylaxis.

Other laboratory investigations

Some centres perform other tests of immune function, for example β_2 microglobulin, but these are of doubtful prognostic value.

For those on zidovudine, a monthly full blood count is recommended; this invariably shows marked macrocytosis. Every three months or so it is prudent to arrange serum creatine kinase, as this may be raised in the few who develop a myopathy due to the drug.

Anyone on oral ketoconazole should undergo regular tests for liver function. Hepatitis with this drug is rare, but should not be missed.

References

1. Lange, J. M., de Wolf, F., and Goudsmit, J. (1989). Markers for progression in HIV infection. *AIDS*, **3**, suppl. 1, 1513-60.

9 Treatment and prophylaxis

Can AIDS be treated?

It is still a widely-held view that there is no treatment for AIDS. In the sense that 'there is no cure for cancer' this is certainly true; but, like cancer, AIDS encompasses a large number of diseases. Since the earliest recognition of the syndrome there have been treatments available for some of the associated infections and tumours, and the number of these is rapidly increasing.

We are now able to monitor immune function much more accurately, and prevent, diagnose, and treat opportunistic infections more effectively. This has measurably improved the length and quality of the lives of people with HIV and AIDS,[1] a fact which has to be appreciated by clinicians and patients alike if maximum benefit is to be obtained.

Furthermore, there is an increasing number of anti-retroviral agents which have been shown to inhibit the activity of HIV.[2]

Management of serious opportunistic infections

Management of serious opportunistic infections is normally instituted by the hospital, and this book is not the place for detailed discussion of their management. However it is useful for the GP to know something about those treatments that are currently available. Patients may well ask the GP

about in- or outpatient treatments; they will usually be
discharged on these drugs; and occasionally a patient at
home will elect not to be admitted but may want active
treatment.

PCP is the commonest opportunistic infection affecting
people with AIDS, and is eminently treatable with a variety
of regimes, including co-trimoxazole, pentamidine, and a
number of other antibiotics and anti-protozoal agents. Early
diagnosis greatly improves outcome.

Other relatively frequent opportunistic infections for
which treatment is available include cerebral toxoplasmosis, cryptococcal meningitis, *Herpes zoster* and *simplex*
infections, cytomegalovirus retinitis, and mycobacterial
infections.

Most patients treated for these conditions will require
preventive or maintenance treatment, which will often be
continued indefinitely; and this is where the GP is likely to
be involved.

The majority of prophylactic regimes involve oral medication, and should present no difficulty for the GP. However,
PCP prophylaxis with nebulized pentamidine and intravenous maintenance for patients with CMV retinitis will not
be familiar to most practices, and these are therefore discussed in some detail.

Nebulized pentamidine

Following an episode of PCP, many patients are advised to
continue with nebulized pentamidine to prevent further
attacks. The standard regime is pentamidine isethionate
300 mg in 3 ml water inhaled via a nebulizer fortnightly,
normally preceded by a beta-agonist such as nebulized
salbutamol to prevent bronchospasm.

A number of centres are now able to lend the patient a
nebulizer for use at home, obviating the need for fortnightly

visits to hospital. The patient will have been instructed in the use of the nebulizer, which is different from those used for other conditions. Pentamidine is prescribable on the drug tarif, but is expensive, so it is advisable to inform the FHSA if you are going to prescribe the drug: there is no need to identify the patient.

Most patients find inhaling pentamidine for 20–30 minutes rather unpleasant, as it has a bitter taste, and may cause severe coughing. A clear explanation of its importance usually satisfies the patient. Some find it easier to inhale the drug for a few minutes at a time, with frequent breaks, and it is a good idea to have some sweets handy to suck.

Maintenance treatment for *Cytomegalovirus* (CMV) retinitis

CMV retinitis rapidly causes blindness, and, although early treatment is often effective, maintenance therapy is usually recommended to prevent further visual loss.

Maintenance after treatment is normally with ganciclovir (DHPG), which must be given intravenously. A common regime is 5 mg/kg daily on five days a week (Mon.–Fri.). Patients are discharged with either a central Hickman line or a Portacath *in situ*, and the patient or a friend or relative will have been instructed in its use. The infusion takes up to an hour. Aseptic technique is of the utmost importance, and it is advisable for the community nurse to supervise the first few administrations at home. The GP is likely to be asked to prescribe sterile dressing packs, sterile water and so on; but the drug itself will be provided by the hospital.

Problems with infection and blockage of the line may be managed by the GP; but if there is any doubt at all, the patient should be referred back to the ward or clinic.

Monitoring for myelosuppression will normally be arranged by the hospital.

Minor infections

Management of **minor infections** is likely to be in the hands of the GP. The difference with the HIV-positive patient is that follow-up should be earlier, as the following example illustrates.

Roger had been HIV-positive for at least five years, and had not experienced any serious illness. He came to surgery extremely anxious one morning, as he had had minor flu symptoms for a few days, with sweating, malaise, and a sore throat, and was now coughing badly without producing any sputum. He denied shortness of breath on exertion, and had not lost any weight.

On examination, his temperature was 38.5° C, and there was some erythema of the soft palate, but no oral hairy leukoplakia or thrush. He did not demonstrate tachypnoea, and his chest sounds were normal.

In the absence of any signs of immune deficiency, the GP was able to reassure both Roger and himself that this was no more than a mild flu-like illness. He advised rest and plenty of fluids, and aspirin or paracetamol if required, and arranged to see Roger again in three days' time, or earlier if he felt worse or developed shortness of breath.

At the follow-up appointment, Roger felt much the same, but was producing small amounts of white and yellow sputum. His temperature was now normal, but there were a few scattered crepitations in both lungs. Roger was again reassured, and at the second follow-up appointment a few days later he had recovered completely.

Some doctors might advocate the use of a broad-spectrum antibiotic in Roger's case, although it is likely that this was a viral infection. Co-trimoxazole should be avoided, as it can partially treat incipient PCP, and delay diagnosis.

These minor upper respiratory tract infections are often a cause of great concern to the patient with HIV, although the majority will resolve spontaneously. Those with severe immune deficiency may benefit from antibiotic treatment, and this would be advised if there is neutropenia—a common finding in the more immune-deficient patient. Any minor infection that does not resolve rapidly should be referred.

Dry, itchy skin is often a problem, and frequent applications of a non-lanolin-based emollient, such as Diprobase®, can give substantial relief. For those with more resistant pruritus, an antifungal cream or ointment with low-strength hydrocortisone, such as Daktacort®, used sparingly, may be useful.

Oral, oesophageal, and vaginal thrush may respond to topical treatment, but oral therapy is usually more effective, although it may have to be maintained indefinitely. Keto-conazole (Nizoral®) is cheaper than the newer oral anti-fungals, but liver function must be monitored regularly. Remember that thrush is a very useful indicator of immune function (see Chapter 7), so treatment is probably best started by the hospital clinic.

Oral acyclovir (Zovirax®) is useful to treat and prevent recurrent herpes infections, and is extremely well tolerated. The dose can be adjusted according to response.

Costs of treatment

Some of these drugs are expensive, but Family Health Services Authorities (FHSAs) have made it clear that if a GP informs them of patients on expensive drugs—and there is no need to identify the patient by name—their drug costs will be allowed for in setting indicative budgets.

Prevention of infections

Advice about general hygiene, preparation of food, etc. is dealt with in Chapter 14.

Chemical prophylaxis is an important means of preventing certain serious opportunistic infections, and improvements in this field are having a significant effect on the survival of people with HIV.

The commonest opportunistic infection is PCP. In those with a T-helper count of below 200, there is a 30 per cent chance of developing PCP within a year.[3] There is increasing evidence that prophylaxis against this protozoal infection is effective.

Secondary prophylaxis (i.e. for those who have recovered from one episode of PCP) is now widely offered—some centres feel it should be mandatory for all patients—and may take the form of nebulized pentamidine given fortnightly at home or in the clinic, oral co-trimoxazole in a variety of doses, or dapsone/pyrimethamine or other antiprotozoal agents once a week or more frequently.

The problem with nebulized pentamidine is that it is extremely caustic, and some patients are unable to tolerate it. Bronchospasm is common, and salbutamol is normally given via the nebulizer before the pentamidine. There is some evidence that the lung apices are not reached by the aerosol, and *Pneumocystis* infection has been described in other organs.

Oral prophylaxis can cause allergy and sensitivity, and this can be of significance if the drug is later needed for treatment.

Primary prophylaxis is a more contentious issue, as the risks from prophylaxis have to be weighed against the risk of developing PCP. Many centres offer primary prophylaxis to those with T-helper counts persistently below 200, especially if HIV Ag is persistently raised, even in the absence of clinical immune deficiency.

The patient should also be considered, bearing in mind the disruption caused by taking pills or administering nebulized pentamidine, with their constant reminder of sickness.

Anti-retroviral

The only anti-retroviral drug currently licensed in the UK is zidovudine (azidothymidine, AZT, Retrovir®), although others are available in some clinics on a trial basis.

Zidovudine is a DNA chain terminator, and a competitive inhibitor of reverse transcriptase, an enzyme used by HIV in replication. It has considerable *in vitro* activity against HIV, and *in vivo* a number of studies have shown that, in patients with past PCP infection or severe symptomatic HIV infection, the drug significantly reduces mortality and morbidity and the number of episodes of opportunistic infection.[4,5]

However, side-effects can be a serious problem with zidovudine, the commonest being myelosuppression, which is generally more marked in those with low T-helper counts. At the recommended dose of 1200 mg daily up to 40 per cent of patients develop anaemia,[6] often severe enough to require blood transfusion. However, many centres are now using lower doses, a policy which greatly reduces this problem, and appears to have little effect on the benefits derived from the drug, although there is concern that CNS levels may be too low to prevent the effects of HIV on the CNS.

There is evidence that the benefits of zidovudine in patients with symptomatic HIV disease do not last indefinitely,[7] and this causes difficulties in judging the optimal time to use it.[8]

A large study is under way looking at the benefits of giving zidovudine to those with asymptomatic HIV infection.

Which patients should be offered zidovudine?

Expert opinion varies, from those who recommend the drug to anyone with HIV infection whose T-helper count is below 400, to those who would only recommend it to patients who have had an opportunistic infection, or who have serious HIV disease and a T-helper count below 200. The feelings of the patients should always be considered, and they should always make an informed choice, on the basis of all the information currently available. In HIV-related thrombocytopenia, and HIV-related encephalopathy, zidovudine is the treatment of choice.

The GP can have an important role in the supervision of patients on zidovudine. Once a patient is stabilized on the drug, monthly full blood counts should be performed, and it is quite appropriate for the GP to arrange this. Many patients prefer to attend the GP rather than the hospital every month.

Complementary therapy

As with any disease, it is of great benefit for patients to understand and be in control of their own management. From the early days of the epidemic, it was apparent that some patients did much better than others, particularly those who took a positive outlook and involved themselves in decision-making. A high proportion of patients with HIV have used some form of complementary therapy (Westminster hospital, personal communication); and, while controlled studies in this field are probably impossible, as long as the therapy does no harm, patients should be supported.

The future

There is every reason to be hopeful about the future management of HIV disease. Our understanding of the virology of HIV, and its effects on the immune system, have increased rapidly, as has our skill at preventing and treating serious infections.[1]

A number of new anti-retroviral drugs are undergoing trials,[2] and there is important research into the modulation of the immune system. Some experts have predicted that within the next few years it may be possible to control HIV infection successfully, putting it on a par with diabetes or epilepsy.

Immunization to prevent HIV infection is less likely to be successful, at least in the foreseeable future, as the virus changes its genetic make-up so frequently.

Whether the education of the public will ever succeed in preventing new infection remains to be seen; but on current experience this seems extremely unlikely.

References

1. Peters, B. S., Beck, E. J., Coleman, D. G., Wadsworth, M. J. H., McGuinness, O., Harris, J. R. W., and Pinching, A. J. (1991). Changing disease patterns in patients with AIDS in a referral centre in the United Kingdom: the changing face of AIDS. *British Medical Journal*, **302**, 203–7.
2. Palca, J. (1991). The growing anti-HIV armamentarium. *Science*, **253**, 263.
3. Lange, J. M., de Wolf, F., and Goudsmit, J. (1989). Markers for progression in HIV infection. *AIDS*, **3**, suppl. 1, 1513–60.
4. Fischl, M. A. *et al.* (1987). The efficacy of azidothymidine (AZT) in the treatment of patients with AIDS and AIDS-related complex. *New England Journal of Medicine*, **317**, 185–91.
5. Fischl, M. A. *et al.* (1990). The safety and efficacy of zidovudine

(AZT) in the treatment of subjects with mildly symptomatic HIV infection. A double-blind, placebo-controlled trial. *Annals of Internal Medicine*, **112**, 727-37.

6. Richman, D. D. *et al.* (1987). The toxicity of azidothymidine in the treatment of patients with AIDS and ARC. *New England Journal of Medicine*, **317**, 192-7.
7. Fischl, M. A. *et al.* (1989). Prolonged zidovudine therapy in patients with AIDS and advanced AIDS-related complex. *Journal of the American Medical Association*, **262**, 2405-10.
8. Swart, A. M., Weller, I., and Darbyshire, J. H. (1990). Early HIV infection: to treat or not to treat? *British Medical Journal*, **301**, 825-6.

10   Professional aspects

Confidentiality

Confidentiality is a primary requirement if we are to provide effective care for those affected by HIV. Perceived lack of confidentiality has been shown to be one of the main reasons those with HIV fail to use the primary care services.[1-3]

The public knows that GPs can be asked to provide information about them to a third party, but many do not know that this can only be given with their express written consent.[4]

It is a good idea to have a clear written practice policy on confidentiality, and it would be useful to give a copy to all patients, or enclose the policy with the practice leaflet. The principle should be that no information whatsoever about a patient will be revealed to a third party without their express written permission. Confidentiality should include everyone working in the practice.[5]

The written policy should include details of the disciplinary action that will be taken against any member of staff who breaches confidentiality.

Record-keeping

Without accurate records, we can also fail to provide our patients with effective care, so a useful balance has to be found between keeping proper records and maintaining confidentiality.

Any information of a sensitive nature should be discussed with the patient, and recorded only in a manner acceptable to them. It is helpful to explain the importance of accurate records, and to stress their confidential nature. Once this is made clear, most patients are happy for any information to be written down.

However, if a patient does not want his or her HIV status noted, a code can be used, which is understood only by those working in the practice. Again, this should be discussed with the patient, who should be told who will understand the code. If patients decide on coding of the notes, or that nothing at all should be written down, they should be told how important it is to remind you, or your colleagues, or any other doctor they consult, that they are HIV-positive.

Any information kept on computer should be dealt with similarly.

Insurance companies

We cannot serve two masters.[6] Either we act in the interests of our patients, or of insurance companies, but not both. Most patients do not know what they are consenting to when they sign the bottom of an insurance form.[4] For this reason, it is reasonable to ask to see any patient for whom a request for information has been received, so that you can go through the form with them and explain any difficulties.

Much that appears on these forms is a matter of conjecture (for example 'Is the patient temperate in his habbits?'), and many companies still persist in asking whether the patient is at risk of HIV infection.

One response is either to bracket the 'lifestyle' questions, asking the company to approach the patient direct for the answers, or to return the form to the company with a covering letter, explaining that you do not complete these forms for any patients, but that you are willing to do a full medical, for which your fee is . . . In this case, you should also write to the patient explaining that in view of the conjectural and private nature of some of the questions, there is a practice policy that none of these forms are completed, but that you have offered to do a medical instead. Some patients are angry at the delay involved, for example in obtaining a mortgage or life insurance; but most are pleased that you clearly have their interests at heart. Again, a clear practice policy here is essential.

Communication

Good communication between hospital and general practice is as important in dealing with HIV-positive patients as with any others; yet in practice communication is often far from adequate.[5,7] As GPs we never refer a patient to hospital, whether as an emergency or as an outpatient, without a letter of referral. But how often have you been faced with a patient who has just been seen in an outpatient facility or discharged from hospital, with no communication whatsoever?

This might happen less if all hospital doctors were required to spend part of their training in general practice; but until this happens, we should take every opportunity to teach the hospitals the importance of a useful exchange of information.

With the HIV-positive patient, hospitals have been particularly reluctant to communicate, partly to respect patient confidentiality, and partly because they have doubted the ability or willingness of GPs to be usefully involved in their care.

David was discharged from the ward one Friday afternoon with an indwelling Portacath, through which he had learned to administer DHPG twice a day, aimed at preventing further blindness from CMV retinitis. On the next day, a Saturday, the GP was called in, as David was having difficulty with this Portacath. He was in a state of great anxiety, as he could not get the needle through the subcutaneous diaphragm, and was terrified that he would rapidly become totally blind.

The GP had never seen or heard of a Portacath, but remembered that one of the district nurses had worked on the ward with HIV patients recently; being on duty that morning the nurse was able to come in and show David and his GP what the problem was.

A phone call from the ward when David was discharged would have saved everyone a great deal of stress.

Some clinics have adopted the use of 'shared care' cards, on the model of antenatal clinic cards, which are kept by the patient and completed by hospital doctors and the GP.[8] If the patient is well motivated, and not concerned about the card falling into the wrong hands, these can work well.

Communication by letter is traditional, and also works well, but is dependent on the hospital's understanding the importance of such letters. A brief note from a clinic doctor, handed by the patient to the GP, or vice versa, is much better than nothing. The telephone is also a useful means of communication, and a brief word over the phone about a patient can be extremely useful.

Discharge letters on a standard form could be issued to all patients on discharge, to be handed personally to the GP.

Effective communication within the primary care team is essential—regular meetings assist this, and the relatively small number of people involved facilitates rapid and effective informal communication.

Infection control

Control of infection in the clinical context means avoiding transmission of HIV through inoculation with used 'sharps', and the avoidance of contamination of broken skin or mucous membranes with infected body fluids.

- **Sharps** should *never* be re-sheathed, but disposed of in a sharps bin, which should be within easy reach whenever sharps are used.
- Any **cuts or abrasions** should be covered with a waterproof dressing.
- **Spillages of body fluids** should be covered with Presept granules and wiped up, using gloves, with paper towels.
- **If hands are contaminated** with body fluids *from any patient*, they should be washed immediately with Hibiscrub or Betadine, or plenty of soap if these are not available.
- **Protective clothing** (latex gloves and plastic aprons) should be worn when the carer is exposed to blood or

body fluids *from any patient*, and these items of clothing should be discarded after use.

- **Masks and eye protection** are only necessary when there is significant risk of infected body fluids entering the eyes.

- **Clinical waste** should be disposed of in suitable plastic bags, which many local authorities provide and will collect.

- **Washing of soiled clothing** and other material presents no problem, as a hot wash with plenty of detergent destroys HIV.

Some authorities now recommend prophylactic treatment with zidovudine following needlestick injury involving body fluid known to be infected with HIV. Treatment should be commenced if possible within an hour of injury, and accident forms should be completed.

The risks of acquiring infections other than HIV from a patient are minimal. There is the possibility of transmission of tuberculosis and CMV; but most health care workers are immune to the former, and have probably already been exposed to the latter. It should be emphasized that it is a patient's immune deficiency that allows infections which are normally virtually harmless to cause serious disease, and that most of these opportunistic pathogens are already being carried by most of us.

The primary care team

Experience has demonstrated that the primary care team is well equipped to care for those of us in the community affected by HIV.[8] It is desirable to draw on the skills of GPs, district nurses, practice nurses, health visitors, clinical nurse specialists, physiotherapists, occupational therapists, social workers, home helps, community care assistants, and any other community health care workers as appropriate.

Where a large number of workers are involved, it is useful to have one key worker, so that work is not duplicated, and so that patients have every opportunity to have their needs met. The key worker may be the GP, or any other member of the team. Grant's situation is a good example of the interactions between patients and carers.

Grant had recently been discharged following treatment for Leishmaniasis, PCP, and CMV retinitis, the last of which had caused complete blindness in one eye and for which he was receiving daily DHPG through a Hickman line. He also had a number of Kaposi's sarcoma lesions, and oral thrush. He had lost a lot of weight, and had decided to remain at home.

His daughter had nursed her mother until her death from cancer, and was understandably concerned about going through a similar experience with her father.

The district nurses made daily visits, as did the physiotherapist and occupational therapist. However, his community care assistant developed a particularly close relationship with Grant and his daughter, and in fact became the key worker, as she best understood what they wanted. Grant eventually died very peacefully and comfortably in his own bed, with his family and friends around him.

Reception staff

The role of receptionists is often underestimated, but they are the interface between the primary care team and the public. A good receptionist helps the patient to make best use of the services available, and is invaluable in the efficient running of the practice. The receptionist should have clear guidelines on practice policy concerning registration of new patients, and on dealing with those who are on the list.

All reception staff should understand the importance of confidentiality, particularly where sensitive information is concerned. Given clear guidelines, a good receptionist can provide an excellent service to patients with or affected by HIV.

Practice policy

There should be a clear practice policy on the following issues:

- **confidentiality**
- **injecting drug users**
- **patients with HIV**
- **provision of safe behaviour advice**
- **provision of condoms**
- **provision of needles and syringes.**

References

1. Helbert, M. (1987). AIDS and medical confidentiality. *British Medical Journal*, **295**, 552.
2. King, M. (1988). AIDS and the general practitioner: views of patients with HIV infection and AIDS. *British Medical Journal*, **297**, 182–4.
3. Mansfield, S. J. and Singh, S. (1989). The general practitioner and human immunodeficiency virus infection: an insight into patients' attitudes. *Journal of the Royal College of General Practitioners*, **39**, 104–5.
4. Lorge, R. E. (1989). How informed is patients' consent to release of medical information to insurance companies? *British Medical Journal*, **298**, 1495–6.
5. King, M. (1987). AIDS and the general practitioner: psychosocial issues. *Health Trends*, **19**, 1–3.

6. Toon, P. and Jones, E. (1986). Serving two masters: a dilemma in general practice. *Lancet*, **i**, 1196-8.
7. Smits, A., Mansfield, S., and Singh, S. (1990). Facilitating care of patients with HIV infection by hospital and primary care teams. *British Medical Journal*, **300**, 241-3.
8. George, R. and Moss, A. (1991). AIDS—the impact on primary care. In *The Medical Annual*, (ed. J. Fry and T. Bouchier Hayes), pp. 15-21. Clinical Press Ltd, Bristol.

11   Psychological aspects

The primary care team

Dealing with the terminally ill, the chronically sick, and people with life-threatening conditions brings particular difficulties for the primary care team. When those affected are young it can be particularly stressful. Even those with HIV who are well are often subject to severe anxiety at times, and it can be hard for the team to deal with this.

Some psychological support for all the members of the team is essential. For health authority staff this may be already in existence, with managers supervising and supporting those under their authority. If such support is not available, it should be discussed with the managers concerned, and arranged. However, for the self-employed GP such support is all too often lacking, and the GP may not be aware of this need.

For the GP, help may be available from partners or other colleagues; but, if not, it is important to find someone who is willing to be available on a regular or informal basis, to whom the GP can express anxieties and causes of stress.

Regular communication within the team is essential, and should be arranged so that all those present feel able to talk freely about any problems, whether with patients or with their own coping mechanisms. It can be particularly useful to have access to an impartial 'facilitator', such as a community psychiatric nurse. Any problems should be dealt with quickly, as unresolved conflicts within the team affect the delivery of adequate care.

All those working in the HIV field should have examined their own attitudes to confidentiality, HIV, drug-users, sexuality, and death, as these issues crop up frequently, and only by being aware of our own attitudes can we cope effectively.

Friends, family, informal carers

The psychological stress on those close to anyone affected by HIV, particularly if the patient is very ill, can be immense. It is essential that all those involved should have opportunities to express their feelings and fears, whether to each other, to voluntary workers, or to members of the primary care team. Often all that is required is a simple explanation of what is going on, and straightforward replies to any questions.

Particularly around the dying, strong emotions frequently surface, and these may appear to be seriously misdirected. However, such emotions must be expressed, as they can cause intolerable strain on the patient and everyone else.

One dying patient was particularly fond of smoking cannabis, and one day one of the community nursing sisters found a care assistant rolling a joint for him, as he was blind, and unable to do this himself. The nurse made a complaint to the care assistant's manager, and a great deal of ill feeling was created. However the patient himself rang the nurse's manager and explained that in his situation what had happened was perfectly acceptable, and the matter was resolved amicably.

The patient

Just as for the members of the primary care team and for friends, family, and other carers, it is important for the person with HIV to have every opportunity to express fears and anxieties. The GP should make it clear to all such patients that nothing is too trivial to be mentioned. It may be appropriate to refer a particularly anxious patient for counselling; but most matters can be dealt with by the GP through frank and open discussion.

Many of those with HIV will know a number of others with the virus, and may indeed have lost friends, family, or lovers. The distress this can cause should never be underestimated. Patients often compare themselves with others who have been in apparently similar situations, and in this case it is important to stress that everyone is different.

Maintenance of a realistic but positive outlook is essential—there are many reasons for someone with HIV to be increasingly optimistic.

An important factor in those who have survived many years with HIV appears to be the degree of understanding and control of their own management demonstrated by the people affected. At all times the GP should explain frankly what is going on, what treatment is being offered, and why, so that patients have maximum control of their own management. Indeed, a survey in New York of long-term survivors with AIDS showed that the majority had fired at least one doctor!

Self-help groups and the newsletters published by them are a very useful source of information about HIV and AIDS, and provide a point of contact for those affected. Isolation can be very distressing, but some patients require persuasion to take up the services offered. Every part of the country has groups and organizations providing information and support for people affected by HIV, and every health district has an AIDS co-ordinator, often based at the GUM clinic, who will know what local services are available (see Chapter 18).

The worried well

There is a group of patients who repeatedly request HIV antibody tests, but who are repeatedly HIV antibody negative. They have become known as 'the worried well', and can become very demanding, utilizing scarce counselling resources.

Managing such patients is not new to GPs, who are used to frequent attenders who have no serious physical illness. The principles are to give the patients an opportunity to express their anxieties freely, to provide as much reassurance as possible, to look for features of anxiety, depression, and obsessional disorders, and to refer if necessary.[1]

References

1. Miller, D. (1987). Counselling. In *ABC of AIDS*, (ed. M. W. Adler), pp. 37–40. British Medical Journal, London.

12 Social aspects

Injecting drug-users

There is a general perception among GPs that injecting drug-users are dishonest, unreliable, and chaotic in their behaviour.[1] This is debatable, as the service offered to them is often inferior to that provided for others. Few areas have a satisfactory back-up service for the GP providing care for drug-users, and this exacerbates the problem. However, it is useful to have a practice policy for dealing with this group. Some practices will provide general medical services to those already on the list, and may or may not be prepared to issue prescriptions for controlled drugs.

A practice policy about taking on new patients who seek prescriptions for controlled drugs or drugs liable to abuse is essential.

Having identified those who are injecting drugs, it is reasonable to provide them with sterile needles and syringes, either on demand, or on an exchange basis. At the very least, you should let them know where clean works are available. The importance of correct use of needles and syringes should be stressed at every opportunity, as well as the importance of safe sex.

Housing

Adequate housing is a necessity for people with HIV, as they are at risk of life-threatening infections, diarrhoea, breathing difficulties, and weakness, and good nutrition is essential.

Ideally housing should be self-contained, with adequate facilities for storage and preparation of food, and with level access from the street.

Some housing authorities have a specific policy on the housing of people with HIV,[2] although each case is normally dealt with on individual merit. Local housing departments can advise about their particular policy, if any.

Social workers can be very useful in pushing for adequate housing, and back-up evidence from the GP and hospital doctor can be very helpful. A phone call to the housing officer concerned can work wonders, although any communication should only ever be with the express, and preferably written, permission of the patient.

Benefits

State benefits are generally tailored to individual means and needs, although mobility allowance and attendance allowance (or terminal care allowance) are not means-tested. Benefits apply generally to the individual's specific needs, rather than to a specific diagnosis. Someone with AIDS who is perfectly well may not be entitled to any state benefits, while someone with symptomatic HIV infection may qualify for a number of benefits. Social workers should be asked to help patients claim whatever they are entitled to. In some areas there are social workers who specialize in the needs of people with HIV.

Employment

The decision to tell an employer that an employee is HIV+ must remain with the individual. It may be totally irrelevant, and many employers are still ignorant about the issues around HIV. However, for those who need time off work from time to time, for example to attend the clinic, it can be helpful to confide in one colleague, providing confidentiality is maintained.

An exception is those whose work puts them at risk of infecting others, for example dentists and surgeons. For these people, there are recommendations from their governing bodies, which state in essence that it is an individual's responsibility to discuss the matter with an expert, whose advice should be taken.

Practical issues around death

Government guidelines stipulate that anyone who has died with AIDS should be placed in a body bag. This can be very distressing for friends and carers, so it is best to allow all those who wish to view the body to do so before the funeral directors arrive.

Many undertakers are now used to dealing with people with HIV who have died, and the National Association of Funeral Directors have a clear policy on this. However, not all undertakers follow these guidelines, and it is wise to check out local companies beforehand.

There is no legal requirement to state 'AIDS' on a death certificate, and it is not a notifiable disease. However, for statistical reasons it is helpful to include a diagnosis that is clearly associated with AIDS, or to tick the box on the back of the certificate, stating that the GP will provide further information later if required. If the relatives are particularly anxious about what is written on the death certificate, a vague term such as 'pneumonia' is perfectly acceptable.

Funeral arrangements are not infrequently made by the patient before death, and there is much to commend this. Sometimes no one attends the crematorium or burial, and there is a party, or 'wake', to celebrate the life of the person who has died.

It is particularly important for gay people, and others in stable relationships, to make a will, so that there is no argument about who inherits the estate. Unfortunately it is not unknown for a parent to take the keys from a lover, and refuse any access to the joint home.

References

1. McKegany, N. P. and Boddy, F. A. (1988). General practitioners and opiate-abusing patients. *Journal of the Royal College of General Practitioners*, **38**, 73-5.
2. Smith, S. J. (1990). AIDS, housing, and health. *British Medical Journal*, **300**, 243-4.

3   Children and families

Pregnancy

Current evidence suggests that only about 13 per cent of children born to a mother with HIV will themselves have HIV infection, although most will have HIV antibody for many months.[1] Of those children with HIV infection, a high proportion are likely to develop AIDS—few survive beyond the age of five.

Getting pregnant involves unsafe sex, but the decision to plan a pregnancy must remain with the parents. Couples should be offered all the available information about the risk of HIV transmission to the partner, and to the child, and if one of them is HIV-positive they should consider the possibility that a child may be left without one of the parents.

There is also some evidence that pregnancy can further impair immune function in a woman with HIV infection,[2] and this should be borne in mind.

It is helpful to seek the involvement of the health visitors early on in pregnancy, as well as the midwives.

Children with HIV

Children with HIV infection may present with persistent lymphadenopathy, splenomegaly, and hepatomegaly, and oral candidiasis and parotitis are much more common in HIV-infected children than in children presumed un-infected.[1] Failure to thrive is a common presentation.

By 12 months, 26 per cent of infected children have AIDS, and 17 per cent die of HIV-related disease.[1]

If a parent, particularly the mother, is known to be HIV-positive, it is important to keep a close eye on the child for any signs of HIV disease.

The role of the GP here is no different from that in other cases where a child's health is at risk, and the family needs particular support and supervision. Families affected by haemophilia are such an example. In the following case, it was not known how Mark's mother had acquired HIV.

Mark's mother had remained well during the pregnancy, despite being HIV-positive. He was born at term, rather underweight. He was bottle-fed, and for three or four months presented no problems, remaining at about the fifth centile for weight. According to the hospital, he was HIV antibody positive, but they were unable to say whether he had HIV infection.

The health visitors kept a close eye on him, and soon referred him to the GP when he developed a severe skin rash at about four months. He had a widespread exfoliating erythema, affecting large areas of his trunk and limbs. Mark was referred back to the hospital, who diagnosed a dermatitis, which responded well to topical hydrocortisone.

Both his mother and the GP were extremely anxious about Mark, particularly when his weight fell well below the fifth centile. However, at about ten months the hospital were satisfied that Mark was not infected with HIV, and by the time he was one year old he was developing normally.

Maternal antibody to HIV may persist in a child for many months, even if the child does not have HIV infection; but the hospital clinic may be able to give an indication whether the child is actually infected by monitoring tests of immune function and HIV antigen.

The team will need to offer a great deal of support to a mother in this situation.

Mark's father had been living with his wife when Mark was born, but shortly afterwards left home after a row. He was HIV antibody negative, and neither he nor his wife had ever injected drugs. Mark's mother lost some weight, and had recurrent problems with oral and vaginal thrush, so was started on zidovudine and keto-conazole, as well as PCP prophylaxis. Her main concern was that her neighbours would discover she had HIV infection, and the health visitors and social worker needed considerable discretion about visiting. It took much convincing to persuade her to let Mark go to a nursery three days a week, but once he had started she found she welcomed the free time. She progressed well, and has been hopeful that her husband will move back home.

In families where one or more members are known to be HIV-positive, it is useful, with the consent of the family, to seek the involvement of health visitors and social workers at an early stage. This helps build up trust and confidence, which is important, as it is likely that the family will need increasing support as time goes on. The principles of care are no different from those for any other family affected by chronic illness, and here again the primary care team is well equipped to help; but the specific issues raised by HIV must be understood by everyone involved.

If problems arise at school, one key worker, well acquainted with the facts about HIV, can be invaluable.

Women with HIV

The patterns of disease in women with HIV infection have not been as well studied as in men, but it does appear that the disease has a poorer outcome in women.[3]

Gynaecological problems are particularly troublesome, and cervical cancer can be aggressive in immunocompromised women.[4,5] It is therefore essential for all women with HIV to be offered frequent cervical screening, and offered prompt and thorough treatment where indicated.

Gynaecological problems in women with HIV include:[3]

- Chronic vaginal candidiasis
- Vaginitis
- Colpitis
- Genital folliculitis and dermatitis
- Herpes genitalis
- Cervical atypia
- Chronic pelvic infection
- Ovarian cystic tumour, abscess, carcinoma
- Menstrual abnormalities

Primary health care for all women should be accessible and acceptable, including the provision of family planning services and safe behaviour advice.

References

1. European collaborative study (1991). *Lancet*, **337**, 253–60.
2. Bird, A. and Snow, M. (1988). HIV monitoring of pregnant women. *Lancet*, **i**, 713.
3. Jones, L. and Catalan, J. (1989). Women and HIV disease. *British Journal of Hospital Medicine*, **41**, 526–38.
4. Bradbeer, C. (1987). Is infection with HIV a risk factor for cervical intraepithelial neoplasia? *Lancet*, **ii**, 1277–8.
5. Spurrett, B., Jones, D., and Stewart, G. (1988). Cervical dysplasia and HIV infection. *Lancet*, **i**, 237–8.

14   General health

Diet

It is interesting to note that PCP is seen in malnourished children in the absence of HIV. Clearly nutrition is important in the maintenance of a healthy immune system. Good dietary habits are essential for everyone, but especially for those who may be prone to immune deficiency. Some clinics provide dietitians with a particular interest in the nutrition of those with HIV, and the GP can refer to them, or to generic dietitians.

The basic advice on diet is to encourage a well-balanced, healthy diet, containing appropriate proportions of protein, carbohydrate, and fat, and plenty of vitamins. Patients should be encouraged to eat when they're hungry, not necessarily confining themselves to particular meal-times.

Food hygiene

Particular foods are more likely to contain bacterial contamination, and many with HIV prefer to avoid these—for example eggs, shellfish, poorly cooked meat, etc. Hygiene in the kitchen is essential—for example washing hands thoroughly, washing after handling raw meat, and keeping a separate chopping board for raw meat. Storage of food is also important, and manufacturers' recommendations should be followed. Some prefer not to drink tap water, as occasionally this has been contaminated with *Cryptosporidium*. Apart from standard precautions with food, people with HIV should make sensible decisions that they are comfortable with.

Dietary supplements

For those with chronic diarrhoea, ingestion of essential vitamins and minerals is essential, and it may be necessary to prescribe these specifically. Food supplements can be a useful adjunct for those with anorexia, for example *Fresubin*®, *Hycal*®, *Nutrimel*®, etc.

Some complementary practitioners advocate multivitamin supplements, or bizarre diets—for example, macrobiotic diets. These may suit some patients, and if there is no risk of dietary deficiency, there is no reason to discourage them. However some diets can become very boring, and this may be a disadvantage. It is very difficult to study in a controlled way the effect of particular diets, although many claims are made. Patients should make their own choice about these, and review their own response.

Exercise

Regular exercise will benefit those with HIV just as much as anyone else, because of the physical benefits, as well as its effect on general well-being. It certainly appears that T-helper counts rise in most people after exercise, although whether this is of any importance in the context of HIV infection is not known—but it can hardly do any harm!

Exercise should be matched to the individual's ability and state of health. A good walk, fast enough to cause a little shortness of breath, is probably the best form of exercise, and is available to everyone.

Dental care

Good oral hygiene is essential for anyone with HIV, as this helps maintain appetite and aids digestion. Teeth should be cleaned thoroughly if possible after each meal, and certainly twice a day. The regular use of an antiseptic mouthwash such as Corsodyl® is recommended.

The dentist should be visited regularly. It is best if patients inform the dentist of their HIV status, although the precautions that should be taken by all dentists with all patients should remove any risk of cross-infection in either direction. However, many dentists are still reluctant to treat patients known to have HIV, and if there is difficulty finding a helpful dentist, the local health advisers at the GUM clinic, or the local AIDS co-ordinator should be able to help. If all else fails, the patient can be referred to the local dental department.

Smoking

Advice here is the same as for anyone, but obviously if an individual is at particular risk of chest disease, smoking is unwise. The effect of smoking on susceptibility to tumours is well known, and again is an unnecessary added risk in those with an underfunctioning immune system.

Alcohol

The potentially harmful effects of alcohol should be considered exactly as for everyone else.

Drugs

There is no direct evidence that street drugs have any specific effect on the immune system, but if there is damage to general health, the ability to fight infections may be impaired. One exception would be anabolic steroids, which are subject to abuse, and which can have a direct effect on the immune system.

It is the incorrect use of injectable drugs which puts others at risk of HIV infection, and the user at risk of serious infections such as hepatitis B and septicaemia. Some GPs are uncomfortable with providing users with sterile syringes and needles, and showing users how to sterilize works. However all GPs should be prepared to explain the risks of using unsterile equipment, and know where to refer users for clean works.

Vaccinations

For those with HIV, *live vaccines should be avoided*, unless benefit outweighs risk. Measles and live polio vaccines have however not so far shown any serious complications, but both BCG and smallpox have.[1] Yellow fever vaccine should be avoided if possible.

There is no evidence that immunization accelerates the course of HIV infection. Serological response to most vaccines is reduced in people with HIV, depending on the degree of immunosuppression present.[1]

Killed or attenuated vaccines are safe: indeed it is important that every patient with HIV should be up to date with diphtheria, tetanus, and especially hepatitis B vaccine, as hepatitis B can be particularly virulent in these patients.

Travel

Restrictions on travel which affect those with HIV are imposed by some governments, including the British government. In most cases this affects only those who are going abroad to work or to seek medical treatment. Most travel insurance policies exclude pre-existing conditions, and HIV and AIDS specifically, and this should be borne in mind.

The International Red Cross have stated that they will help people with HIV and AIDS where there are difficulties at airports and so on.

Another factor to remember is the effect of travel on susceptibility to opportunistic infections. We have seen significant numbers of people with symptomatic HIV infection and AIDS who have developed PCP shortly after a long flight. Whether this is due to reduced oxygen levels in the plane, or the effects of tiredness and jet-lag, is not clear.

Appropriate immunizations are advisable, including typhoid and cholera for travellers to endemic areas; and anti-malarial prophylaxis should not be forgotten. As with all travellers, there is no substitute for adequate hygiene and the avoidance of food and drink that may be contaminated.

Pets

Because of the risk of toxoplasmosis, most authorities recommend that people with HIV should not handle cat-litter trays, or should wear gloves if they do.

Psyche

General well-being is essential to maintaining a healthy immune system and promoting health. Stress, anxiety, and unresolved conflicts can impair well-being, and many people with HIV have discovered it gives them the opportunity to examine their lives and relationships and put right things which are causing distress.

A number of voluntary groups provide advice about maintaining psychological, as well as physical, well-being, and many patients find their services invaluable (see Chapter 18).

References

1. von Reyn, C. F., Clements, C. J., and Mann, J. M. (1987). Human immunodeficiency virus infection and routine childhood immunization. *Lancet*, **i**, 669–72.

15 The health needs of gay men

At the current stage of the epidemic in the UK, 79 per cent of AIDS cases and 58 per cent of HIV-positive reports have been among gay men.[1] Much has been written in the medical literature about the specific problems of injecting drug-users and haemophiliacs, but very little on the specific needs of gay men with HIV.

This must be a reflection of the prejudice still directed against gays and bisexuals. Prejudice among GPs has been shown in a number of questionnaires. According to a survey of 73 trainers in the South West Thames Region, 33 per cent said the greatest deterrent to caring for people with AIDS was the homosexual practices of many patients,[2] and in another study 6 per cent of GPs were reluctant to have gays on their lists.[3]

Section 28 of the Local Government Act demonstrated the intense homophobia still present in this society, and was largely a reaction to the public's fear of AIDS and prejudice against gay women and men. Male gay sex is still not *legal* in the United Kingdom, it is merely decriminalized in certain very specific instances. The age of consent for gay men is 21, well above most other Western and Eastern European countries.

However, the gay community has responded in both Europe and the USA in the most positive way to the threat posed by AIDS. Furthermore, there is evidence that the rate of new HIV infection among gay men has dropped remarkably, and is indeed well below that for hetero-sexuals.

Social background

Because of prejudice and discrimination, many gay men have not been open about their sexuality to family, friends, employers, and GPs, and therefore often lack the support in difficult times such as illness and bereavement that others rely on.

Fear of AIDS

Many gay men have lost lovers or friends with AIDS, and many more know of acquaintances or friends of friends who are HIV+, or who have AIDS or have died. There is still a lack of information about the improvements in management. For these reasons, and maybe others, large numbers of gay men who may have been at risk of acquiring HIV do not get tested, and may even ignore symptoms that they are afraid may be due to HIV. The clinics and hospitals are still seeing patients, many of whom have not been tested, presenting seriously ill with rampant PCP or other opportunistic infections, many of whom die very quickly. Statistics suggest that gay men are being tested later than others, and present later.[1]

General health

Hepatitis B immunization should be recommended for all sexually active gay men, as this virus is more infectious than HIV, and may be acquired even if apparently safe sexual practice is being followed.

Legal matters

Until gay relationships are recognized in law, it is essential for all gay partners to make a will, otherwise the deceased's estate will be left to the family, according to statute.

If there are any life policies which were taken out in good faith before the policy holders knew of their HIV status, it is wise to get a solicitor to draw up an affidavit to this effect, in order to avoid difficulties with the insurer.

References

1. PHLS AIDS Centre. Quarterly surveillance tables No. 11, June 1991.
2. Sibbald, B. and Freeling, P. (1988). AIDS and the future general practitioner. *Journal of the Royal College of General Practitioners*, **38**, 500–2.
3. Sibbald, B., Pharoah, C., Freeling, P., and Anderson, H. R. (1988). AIDS—Is general practice meeting the challenge? *Journal of the Royal College of General Practitioners*, **38**, 32.

16   Palliative care at home

Nationally, only 30 per cent of all people die at home, and the majority of people with AIDS still die in hospital.[1,2] In my own practice, over a four-year period we cared for 39 people with AIDS, of whom 9 died in hospital or in a hospice, and 12 died at home. This means that 63 per cent of AIDS-associated deaths were at home.[3]

Ideally, patients and their friends and carers should have the choice as to where death takes place, whether at home, in a hospice, or in hospital. My impression, after talking to many patients about this issue, is that most would prefer to die at home, given the choice.

Their are particular difficulties which arise when dealing with patients dying with AIDS. These relate to the difficulty of deciding just when a patient is actually dying, and balancing palliative care with active intervention.

Michael was HIV-positive, and had cared for his lover who had died some three years previously. He had lost a lot of weight recently, and was barely able to walk. Over a few days he became confused, and unable to get out of bed. He and his friends were understandably unsure whether he should be admitted, as they were afraid that he was dying, in which case they wanted him to remain peacefully at home. The GP explained that he might have a treatable infection, and indeed on admission he was shown to have cerebral toxoplasmosis, which was treated. A year and a half later he remains well, and able to work.

Symptomatology

Symptoms among patients with AIDS admitted for palliative care broadly compare with those for all patients in hospices.[4]

The GP and the primary care team are well equipped to deal with the patient dying at home, and are able to draw on their experience.

The guiding principles should be to offer the patient choices about how and where to die, and to manage symptoms effectively. Consideration should be given to family and friends, and respite care should be offered if available. An increasing number of hospices are now willing to provide respite and palliative care for people with AIDS, and most have a home support team skilled in this work. It is wise to contact the local hospice sooner rather than later, so that problems can be anticipated before they arise.

References

1. Kennedy, A. (1990). Communicable Diseases Surveillance Centre, Public Health Laboratories. (Unpublished.)
2. Smits, A., Mansfield, S., and Singh, S. (1990). Facilitating care of patients with HIV infection by hospital and primary care teams. *British Medical Journal*, **300**, 241-3.
3. Moss, A. (1991). Therapy in the community. In *Care in the community.* All-party Parliamentary Group on AIDS, London.
4. Sims, R. and Moss, V. (1991). In *Terminal care for people with AIDS.* Edward Arnold, London.

17 Conclusions

> No man is an island, entire of itself; every man is a piece of the Continent, a part of the main. Any man's death diminishes me, because I am involved in Mankind; and therefore never send to know for whom the bell tolls; it tolls for thee.
>
> John Donne, 1573–1631

AIDS is everyone's problem.

We are all at risk of HIV, whether through clinical practice or because of other behaviour.

We are all affected by HIV. If we don't already have patients, friends or relatives with the virus, it is likely we soon shall.

But AIDS is also everyone's opportunity. It has provided an opportunity to break down barriers of stigma and prejudice. It has allowed the development of exciting new standards of client-centred care. And it has shown the incredible bravery, and the willingness to fight, of those of us who are affected.

A GP had noticed a strange furry-looking white plaque on the side of his tongue. It was unlike anything he had seen before, but as it was causing no discomfort he ignored it.

A year later, at a lecture for GPs on HIV and AIDS, a slide was shown demonstrating oral hairy leukoplakia, which is virtually pathognomonic of HIV infection. The GP realized this was what was on his tongue, and all the terrible implications.

Four years afterwards, he discovered a small purple nodule on his chin, and by then he had seen enough Kaposi's sarcoma to known what it was.

This particular GP is still working three years later, actively involved in trying to persuade us that we are all affected by HIV.

All the people described in this book are real.

18   Resources

There are many statutory and voluntary organizations that patients and health care workers may find useful. National groups and phonelines are listed here, but there are many local services. These may be found in the telephone directory, or by contacting the local AIDS co-ordinator, or the health advisers at the local GUM clinic.

AIDS Care Education and Training (ACET)
PO Box 1323
London W5 5TF
Tel. 081-840 7879

A Christian organization providing education, training, and practical help for people with HIV (for example, night sitting).

Body Positive
PO Box 493
London W14 0TF
Tel. 071-835 1045

A well-established self-help group run by and for people with HIV. Many local groups and centres. Fortnightly newsletter, free for people with HIV.

British Humanist Association
14 Lamb's Conduit Passage
London WC1R 4RH
Tel. 071-430 0908

The British Red Cross
Beautycare and Cosmetic Camouflage Department
National Headquarters
9 Grosvenor Crescent
London SW1X 7EJ
Tel. 071-235 5454

Excellent professional advice on cosmetic camouflaging. Help with difficulties at points of immigration.

Crusaid
1 Walcott Street
London SW1P 2NG

Provides funds on behalf of people with HIV disease, and gives grants to organizations.

Cruse
Cruse House
126 Sheen Road
Richmond
Surrey TW9 1UR
Tel. 081-940 4818

A national charity with 185 branches which helps with counselling, advice, and social issues around HIV and AIDS. Also provides training in bereavement counselling and publishes a newsletter and a journal.

London Lighthouse
111–117 Lancaster Road
London W11 1QT
Tel. 071-792 1200

A centre with a wide range of facilities for people affected by HIV. Residential respite and palliative care unit, counselling, education, day-care facility, and domiciliary services.

Mainliners
PO Box 125
London SW9 8EF
Tel. 071-274 4000 ext. 354

A self-help group for drug-users and ex-users.

Mildmay Mission Hospital
Hackney Road
London E2 7NA
Tel. 071-739 2331

Hospice and respite care for people with HIV.

National AIDS Counselling Training Unit (NACTU) (South)
St Charles Hospital
Exmoor Street
London W10 6DZ
Tel. 081-968 8514/5

Offers courses on AIDS and HIV. Also NACTU (Midlands) and NACTU (North).

National AIDS Helpline
Tel. 0800 567 123

Advice and information on AIDS and HIV.

National AIDS Manual (NAM)
NAM Publications
Unit 407, The Brixton Enterprise Centre
London SW9 8EJ
Tel. 071-737 1846

An invaluable and unique directory of HIV related services in the UK, including a directory of AIDS and HIV treatments and trials.

National AIDS Trust
14th Floor, Euston Tower
286 Euston Road
London NW1 3DN
Tel. 071-383 4246

National voluntary organization to support voluntary sector responses to AIDS and HIV.

Positive Partners
10 Rathbone Place
London W1
Tel. 071-249 6068

A self-help group for partners of people with HIV.

Positively Women
333 Grays Inn Road
London WC1X 8PX
Tel. 071-837 9705

A self-help group for women affected by HIV.

The Terrence Higgins Trust
52–54 Grays Inn Road
London WC1X 8JU
Tel. 071-831 0330; Helpline 071-242 1010

A well-established organization offering telephone advice and education around HIV.

Bibliography

Adler, M. (ed.) (1991). *ABC of Aids* (2nd edn). British Medical Journal, London.

Farthing, C. *et al.* (1988). *A colour atlas of AIDS and HIV disease* (2nd edn). Wolfe Publishing Ltd, London.

Kramer, L. (1990). *Reports from the holocaust.* Penguin, London.

Mansfield, S. and Singh, S. (1990). *The management of HIV infection in primary care.* British Medical Association Foundation for AIDS, London. (Available free of charge.)

Mindel, A. (1990). *AIDS—a pocket book of diagnosis and management.* Edward Arnold, London.

Parkin, J. and Peters, B. (1991). *Differential diagnosis in AIDS.* Wolfe, London.

Pratt, R. (1991). *AIDS: a strategy for nursing care* (3rd edn). Edward Arnold, London.

Sims, S. and Moss, V. (1991). *Terminal care for people with AIDS.* Edward Arnold, London.

Youle, M., Clarbour, J., Wade, P., and Farthing, C. (1988). *AIDS therapeutics in HIV disease.* Churchill Livingstone, Edinburgh.

HIV and AIDS in the community. Available free of charge from the publisher, The All-Party Parliamentary Group on AIDS. Tel. 071-219 5761.

Glossary

acquired immune deficiency syndrome (*see* **AIDS**)
AIDS (acquired immune deficiency syndrome) Serious disorder of the immune system in an individual with, or presumed to have, HIV infection, which is defined by any of a large number of opportunistic infections and tumours, for example *Pneumocystis carinii* pneumonia and Kaposi's sarcoma.
AIDS-related complex (*see* **ARC**)
ARC (AIDS-related complex) Includes a number of conditions due to immune deficiency in an individual with, or presumed to have, HIV infection, but which do not fulfil the criteria for AIDS. For example, night sweats, weight loss, oral candidosis, shingles, oral hairy leukoplakia.
anaemia Deficiency of red blood cells and/or their ability to carry oxygen.
antibody Chemical produced by the body to help fight off a specific infection.
antigen Organism, or part of an organism, present in the bloodstream or tissues.
AZT (*see* **zidovudine**)
Candida albicans **(monilia, thrush)** Fungus which may colonize the mouth, gut, vagina, and other organs, particularly in the presence of immune deficiency. The infection is known as candidosis, moniliasis, or thrush.
CD4+ cells (*see* **T-helper cells**)
cervical cancer Cancer of the cells lining the small passage from the vagina into the womb. Pre-cancerous changes in these cells can easily be detected by smear testing, and if present, treatment is straightforward and

effective. There is evidence that changes in the cervical cells are much commoner in women with HIV infection.

clindamycin Antibiotic effective against a number of organisms, which is sometimes used in the treatment of *Pneumocystis carinii* pneumonia.

CMV (*see* **cytomegalovirus**)

colpitis Inflammation of the lining of the vagina or the neck of the womb.

co-trimoxazole (Septrin®) Antibiotic with a wide range of activity against bacteria and other organisms. First-line therapy for *Pneumocystis carinii* pneumonia.

creatine kinase Chemical released by the liver into the bloodstream in increased amounts when it is damaged.

cryptococcal meningitis Infection of the lining of the brain and spinal cord due to the fungus *Cryptococcus neoformans*, causing headache, neck stiffness, vomiting, and confusion.

cryptosporidiosis Infection due to the parasite *Cryptosporidium muris*, which can cause severe and persistent diarrhoea.

cytomegalovirus (CMV) Virus which many people carry for a lifetime without causing any illness, but which in an individual with immune deficiency may infect the eyes, lungs, gut, and other organs.

cytomegalovirus (CMV) retinitis Infection of the back of the eye due to CMV, which may cause blindness if not treated promptly.

dapsone Drug used to prevent and treat *Pneumocystis carinii* pneumonia. It may also prevent toxoplasmosis.

DHPG (ganciclovir, Cymevene®) Antiviral drug effective against CMV. It has to be given through a drip into a vein.

diazepam (Valium®) Tranquillizer and muscle-relaxant.

dyspnoea Difficulty breathing due to pain or shortness of breath.

ELISA (enzyme-linked immunoabsorbent assay) Method of testing for specific antibodies, e.g. HIV antibody.

Fansidar® Drug containing sulphadoxine and pyrimethamine, which is used to prevent and treat *Pneumocystis carinii* pneumonia. It may also prevent toxoplasmosis.

folliculitis Inflammation of the hair follicles.

ganciclovir (*see* **DHPG**)

genitourinary medicine Branch of medicine dealing with diseases of the genital area, as well as infections that are sexually transmitted.

haemophilia Hereditary disease affecting the ability of the blood to clot.

hepatitis B virus (HBV) Virus which is transmitted through sexual activity or via infected needles. Can cause inflammation of the liver with jaundice.

Hickman line Soft tube leading from a tap on the skin into a vein, through which drugs can be administered.

hepatomegaly Enlargement of the liver.

herpes simplex Virus that causes cold sores on the lips, mouth, face, anus or genital areas.

herpes zoster Virus that causes shingles.

HIV (*see* **human immunodeficiency virus**)

human immunodeficiency virus (HIV) Virus which can damage the immune system, leaving the body open to infections and tumours which are otherwise rare in humans.

HIV antibody Antibody produced by the body in response to the presence of HIV.

HIV antigen Particle of HIV which may be detected in the blood of people with HIV infection.

immunosuppressed/immunocompromised Deficiency in the immune system, causing increased susceptibility to infections and tumours.

Kaposi's sarcoma (KS) Tumour of the lining of small blood vessels, which may occur virtually anywhere in or on the body, and causing pink, red, or purple areas.

ketoconazole (Nizoral®**)** Antifungal drug used to treat thrush and other fungal infections.

lymphadenopathy Swelling of the lymph glands, usually

observed or felt in the neck, armpits, and groins.

Molluscum contagiosum Viral skin infection causing small, pearly, dimpled bumps.

monilia (*see* **candidosis**)

neutropaenia Deficiency of white blood cells, which help in the body's response to infections and tumours.

Nizoral® (*see* **ketoconazole**)

opportunistic infection (OI) Infection caused by an organism which does not normally cause serious illness in someone with a healthy immune system.

oral hairy leukoplakia (OHL) Furry-looking white patch underneath or on the side of the tongue, or inside the cheek.

oral thrush Candidosis affecting the mouth.

parotitis Swelling of the salivary glands below and in front of the ear.

PCP (*see* ***Pneumocystis carinii*** **pneumonia**)

pentamidine Drug given through a vein or inhaled in a fine spray, which is used to prevent and treat *Pneumocystis carinii* pneumonia.

persistent generalized lymphadenopathy (PGL) Swelling of glands in the neck or armpits and associated with HIV infection.

PGL (*see* **persistent generalized lymphadenopathy**)

Pneumocystis carinii **pneumonia (PCP)** Infection of the lungs causing severe malaise, shortness of breath, and a persistent dry cough.

portacath Soft latex tube leading from a reservoir just below the skin into a vein, through which drugs not absorbed by mouth can be administered.

pyrexia Raised body temperature.

pyrimethamine Drug used to prevent and treat *Pneumocystis carinii* pneumonia, which may also prevent toxoplasmosis.

Retrovir® (see **zidovudine**)

retrovirus RNA virus which is able to incorporate itself into the nucleus of a host cell, and make copies of itself.

reverse transcriptase Enzyme which enables HIV to incorporate itself into the DNA in the nucleus of a cell it has infected.

risk behaviour Any behaviour which puts an individual at risk of acquiring or transmitting HIV.

risk groups A redundant term used to describe people deemed to be at particular risk of having or acquiring HIV infection. Everyone is potentially at risk of HIV infection—it is our *behaviour* that puts us at risk.

safe behaviour Behaviour which minimizes the risk of acquiring or transmitting HIV.

safe sex Sexual activity which minimizes the risk of acquiring or transmitting HIV.

salbutamol (Ventolin®) Drug used to dilate the airways in the lungs.

seborrhoeic dermatitis Greasy, flaky inflammation of the skin.

seroconversion The stage at which the body recognizes it has been infected with an organism from outside, and produces antibodies to help fight off the infection.

Septrin® (*see* **co-trimoxazole**)

serum Straw-coloured liquid in which the red, white, and other cells in the blood are carried.

shingles (*see* **herpes zoster**)

splenomegaly Enlargement of the spleen.

T-helper cells (CD4+ cells) One of the types of white blood cells which helps to co-ordinate the immune system's response to infections and tumours. They are a particular target for HIV which may over a period of time cause a dangerous reduction in their numbers and/or ability to work effectively.

tachypnoea Increase in the rate of respiration.

thrombocytopaenia Reduction in the number of thrombocytes, the cells in the blood which are essential for clotting.

thrush (*see* **candidosis**)

toxicity Adverse or harmful reaction to a drug, chemical or organism.

toxoplasmosis Organism which can cause brain abscesses and other infections, particularly in people with immune deficiency.

vaccination Preparation (vaccine) given to someone in order to stimulate their immune system, so that the body is able to recognize and fight off the infection for which the vaccine is specific.

Western blot Electrical method of detecting HIV antibodies in the blood.

zidovudine Drug which interferes with the ability of HIV to reproduce itself, and which has been shown to improve the outcome for many people with ARC and AIDS.

Index